YOGA FOR CHILDREN

YOGA FOR CHILDREN

Esther-Martina Luchs

SEARCH PRESS · LONDON

PAULIST PRESS · NEW YORK
RAMSEY, NJ · TORONTO

First published in 1977 in Great Britain
by Search Press Limited, 2–10 Jerdan Place, London SW6 5PT
and in the USA by Paulist Press
Editorial Office: 1865 Broadway, New York, NY 10023
Business Office: 545 Island Road, Ramsey, NJ 07446
German version published by Wilhelm Goldmann Verlag
Munich, Federal Republic of Germany.

ISBN (UK) 0 85532 376 0
ISBN (USA) 0 – 8091 – 2023 – 2

Library of Congress Catalog Card Number: 77-72468
Printed and bound in Great Britain
by Billing and Sons Limited,
of Guildford, London and Worcester,
for Search Press Limited

Contents

PART ONE

Yoga — health — personality

What is Yoga?

Many people confuse yoga with sensational physical contortions, or imagine it involves lying on a bed of nails or think that it is a religion. Yoga is none of these things. Nor is the headstand yoga, although it *is* a hatha-yoga exercise.

All sorts of peculiar ideas are attributed to yoga. Many years ago, when I came back from my first yoga class full of enthusiasm and told my friends about it, I was astonished to find that they regarded me almost with pity: 'You know, a friend of mine does yoga too. In fact she puts aside one day in the week when she does nothing else and her husband has to look after the baby'. This is the exact opposite of what yoga is supposed to be. A widespread ignorance about yoga has meant that many false and often harmful ideas have been associated with it. But I am convinced that these misconceptions will disappear as more and more people practise true yoga and reap the benefits it has to offer.

So what is yoga? We know that in India from time immemorial men have devoted the greater part of their lives to the acquisition of self-knowledge; to the exploration of human nature and the meaning of existence. They have tried to solve the puzzle: 'who am I?' It has taken endless time and patience to unravel the secrets of existence. Each moment of enlightenment pointed a way forward, the way that led out of suffering: the way of yoga.

Yoga is self-education and control of mind and body, leading to self-knowledge.

Different roads lead to the ultimate goal. Hatha-yoga is one among several systems of yoga that can point the way to perfect health. The aim of all forms of yoga is self-knowledge and a necessary condition of self-knowledge is self-discipline.

The word 'yoga' comes from the Sanskrit and means 'yoke', self-mastery in the sense of complete control of mind and body, and the achievement of perfect mental and physical health.

Our bodies are invigorated by both positive and negative forces of energy and when these are exactly balanced we enjoy perfect health. In Sanskrit the positive energy forces were called *Ha* (which means sun) and the negative forces *Tha* (moon). The word yoga has a double meaning: the first can be roughly translated as 'concurrence' or 'joining together' and the second corresponds to the concept 'yoke'. Hatha-yoga means the understanding of the positive and negative forces of energy and the ability to control them.

We must learn to understand the powers within our own bodies so as to use them correctly and to the full. In this way we can develop our self-awareness and achieve a higher spiritual consciousness. It will be a long and arduous way for anyone who is not already exceptionally fit and supple. But if we want to climb to ever higher spiritual planes we must not allow our bodies to stand in the way.

To climb higher it is not necessary to 'stand on our heads'. The headstand is an excellent hatha-yoga exercise but only for people in good health — and in this instance no one who is over-weight or has bad posture can be considered healthy. We find the headstand and other difficult exercises in practically all books about yoga and we often overlook the fact that only people in good health are advised to attempt them. But who today is completely healthy? Has anyone got a perfectly straight spine and strong back muscles? Many young people today walk and stand badly.

Bad posture apart, not everyone can safely attempt the headstand. The sudden rush of blood to the head can bring on eye and ear ailments in those already predisposed to them, and nobody with abnormally high or low blood pressure should try it. It is senseless to attempt exercises which could damage your health. Someone trying yoga for the first time should do it under expert supervision, at least until he is sure he is not hurting himself. Then he can select exercises suited to his particular needs, which build up his strength and health and overcome his individual weaknesses.

Yoga is based on the principle of *correct* breathing. The combination of breathing and movement improves the circulation and when we move correctly we are led back to the natural right way of breathing without any effort on our part. Who today breathes properly? Even children don't as a rule. We have fallen out of step with nature, alienating ourselves from everything which is the basis of good health and robbing ourselves of our greatest source of strength: calm and quietude. It is not in the

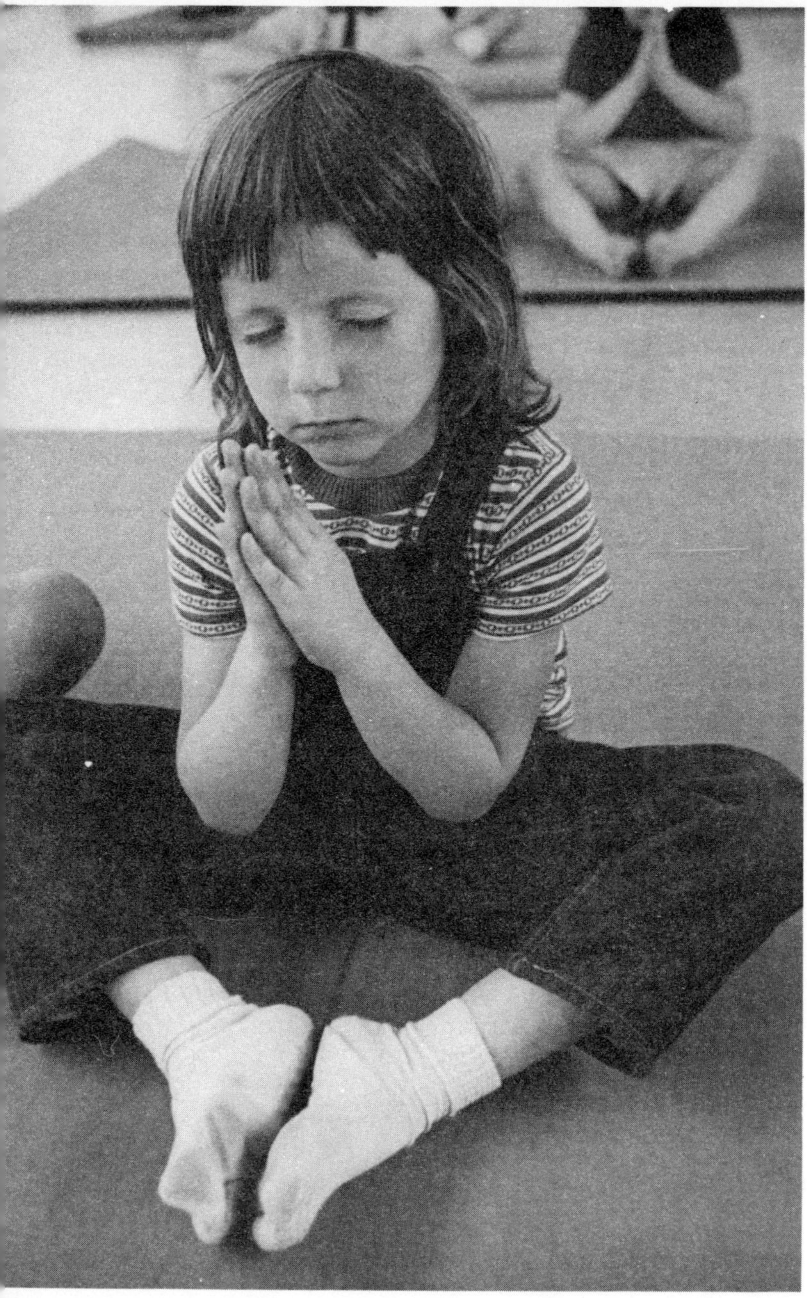

noise and pace of day-to-day existence that we shall find life as we are meant to live it. But yoga exercises (provided we don't try to do too much too soon) will help us to find a way out of the chaos we are caught up in.

Hatha yoga is not gymnastics — quite the contrary: the exercises need nerve-power not muscles. It is not like normal physical training where we expend a great deal of strength and effort: on the contrary, it relaxes and re-charges us with new energy.

Nevertheless, some physical-education teachers and health-farmers try to turn yoga into a competitive sport. That is a waste of energy. The person who turns to yoga is searching for harmony of body, mind and spirit. The whole point of yoga is that it frees people from things that stand in the way of their happiness, and restores to them a lost or broken harmony. It helps us to command our own strength and find ourselves again.

We all know the intimate connexion between mind and body: we know the feeling of being so angry 'it makes our blood boil', of things irritating us and 'getting on our nerves', or of being literally paralyzed by fear. Often people are marked more deeply by mental suffering than by purely physical illnesses.

It is no solution to take our sick bodies to the doctor like a pair of worn-out shoes to the shoe-mender, hoping that he will make us well again. We must also do something to help ourselves. Health is not an unconditional gift; it is our own responsibility. If we are ill it is because the balance between the positive and the negative forces of energy is disturbed. Discontented, dissatisfied and unhappy people fall ill more easily than those who are cheerful, equable, balanced and happy.

Someone who is cheerful and accepts all that life may bring breathes deeply and regularly, whereas someone who is listless and tense takes short shallow breaths. We all know the saying 'take a deep breath and count to ten'; and it is true, for someone who breathes deeply and calmly is in command of the situation and can respond to it positively.

When we are really happy, we breathe deeply and feel outgoing and expansive, as if we could 'hug the whole world'. Fear paralyzes and diminishes us. Observe whether you can breathe deeply and calmly when you are tense and anxious — it's quite impossible. We know too how fear undermines our resistance to illness and increases our vulnerability to infections.

If we want to free ourselves from fear and all its attendant

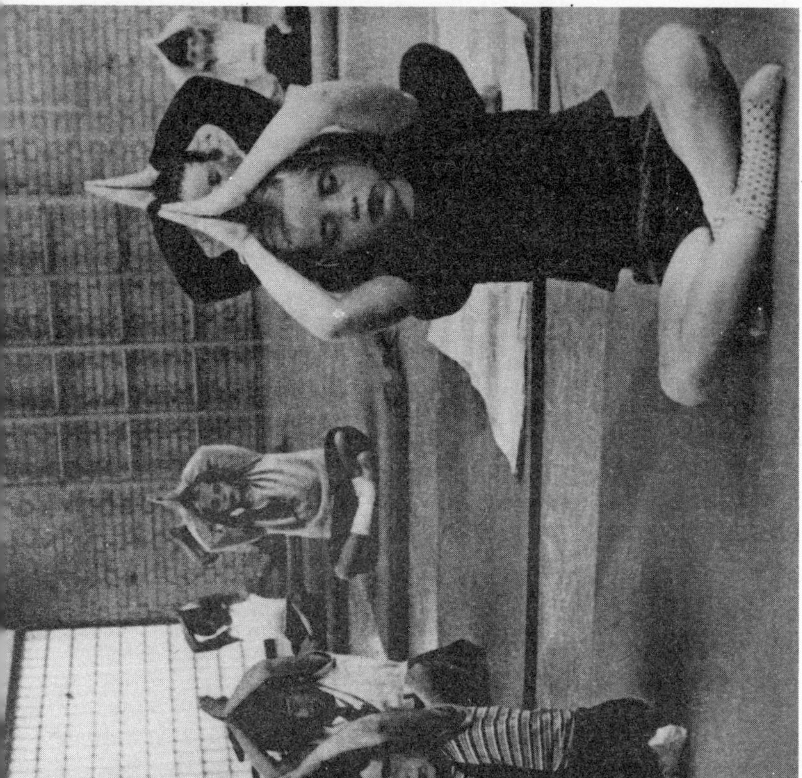

disorders, we must learn to breathe well and deeply again. By breathing wrongly or inadequately we shorten our lives and reduce our energy and zest for life.

To find health, healing and wholeness, we need to master not just our bodies (the way we breathe and move) but also and most important of all, our minds; for the way we think affects not just our health but all aspects of life. To learn to control our thoughts is not easy but the effort is immensely worthwhile. Yoga can teach us how, for it is a unique system comprising the possibilities and prerequisites of a happy life.

Not only adults but children — children especially — need absolute stillness, peace and relaxation. Children are exposed to countless forms of stimulation and, far more than adults, are the unwilling victims of the stress and rush of life today. Our days are so hurried that we no longer find time for a few minutes calm and reflection; they are too full to make room for games and movement; and all too often, a children's playground is a noisy, dusty street. Adults' anxiousness and tension carries over to the children and when, instead of talking to them — offering them understanding, comfort and encouragement — we turn on the television, there is no way they can find the sense of inner peace and belonging they so badly need.

Today a nervous, restless child is no longer an exception, and even quite young children often have horrifyingly bad posture. Children take great pleasure in movement and nothing could provide a better foundation for their continuing good health than hatha-yoga exercises combined with their natural delight in movement. A well-known doctor recommends that children should start yoga when they are five. In his view, no other physical activity (whether physical education, games or athletics) does so much good. Yoga benefits the whole body — internal organs as well as muscles, tendons and spine; it improves children's co-ordination and their ability to concentrate. Nervous children lose their anxiety and develop self-confidence. But he points out that it is important for parents and teachers to be mature and balanced people so that the childrens' trust in the adult world can grow and develop.

Yoga is not a cult or a sect. Rather it is a series of precepts — the rules for physical and spiritual health that can be followed by anyone, irrespective of age or religious beliefs. Yoga is strength, calm and a sense of belonging.

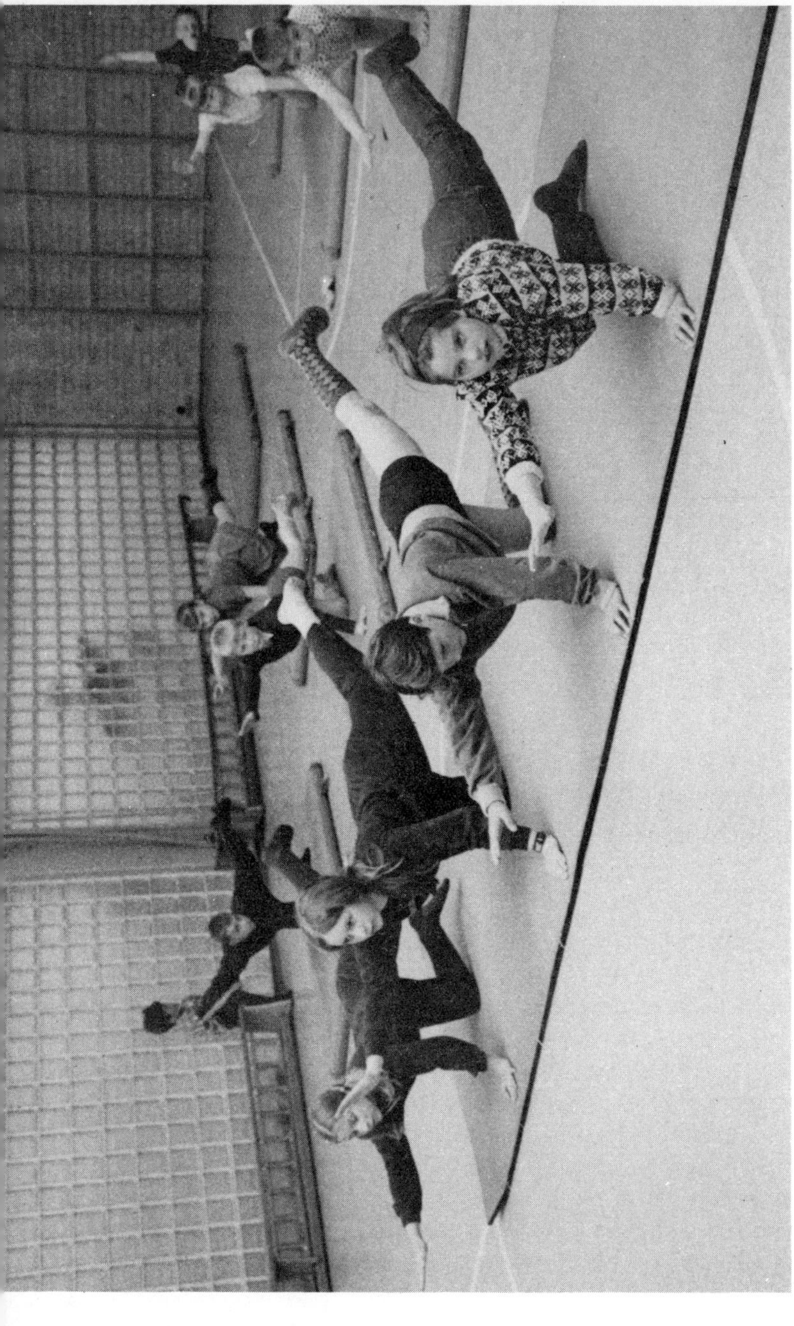

We have not come into the world to be unhappy. It is through an unnatural way of life, not least through civilized living, that man has lost himself. So long as we fail to use our intelligence and to control our thoughts, we shall suffer the consequences. Even the most effective hatha-yoga exercises will not bring us perfect health if we don't build our lives on meaningful foundations, if we don't have enough sleep, if we are one-sided in our concerns, and above all, if we don't eat healthy, nourishing food.

Although we live in a material world — and the things of this world are certainly agreeable — it is not on them that our happiness depends, but on the riches we carry in our hearts.

After many years as a student at Selvarajan Yesudian's and Elizabeth Haich's yoga school, I decided out of gratitude to try to give to others all that I had received there. I hoped that I might succeed in showing those who were tense, irritable and demanding, the way back to an absolute stillness, so that they might find again, at least for a time, what, through the pressure and pace of life, they had lost of their true selves.

Why children should do yoga

Children who can grow up surrounded by the protective love of parents and who have a feeling of security, are not only happier but healthier than those who live under more difficult conditions.

Unfortunately most children today no longer live close to nature and are thus estranged from much that is essential to their health and stability. Life puts so much pressure on children. They lack our defences and have no idea how to protect themselves for they only gradually learn how to build a protective wall against the outside world. Children are so open and truthful, wearing their heart on their sleeve. They have special problems and desperately need an adult's understanding and loving guidance. What they need above all is good health.

For a long time now, young people have been growing up without suffering the hardships of war, and one might assume that they enjoy excellent health. But is this really the case?

Bad posture and general physical weakness have become serious problems. Professor Hans Kraus, John F. Kennedy's doctor, confirms this general impression. In his view, our inactive and over-indulgent way of life is particularly dangerous for children who should be building up strong and supple muscles for their adult years. Children may not often have back-ache, but young people whose muscles are weak and unsupple are lucky to reach their mid or late twenties without suffering something more serious than back-ache. Only very few parents fail to have their children vaccinated against smallpox, polio, diphtheria and other infectious diseases, but how many realize the importance of exercise to children so that they don't develop nervous tension, back-ache and heart disease, or become over-weight, later in life? Illnesses of middle and old age begin in the cradle.

Children today suffer from a serious lack of exercise. Living conditions are cramped and frequently there is no opportunity to play safely near their home. This, and a harrassed mother who hasn't time to take them for a walk in the country or to a children's playground, accustoms them very early in life to an

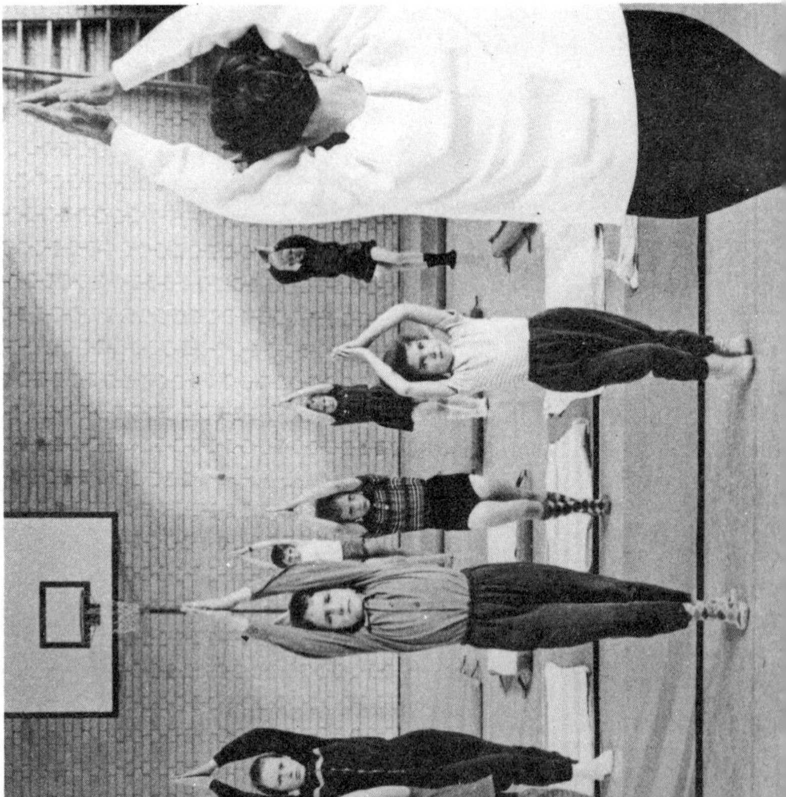

entirely passive existence. In the morning they are taken to school in the car, or they go by bus or train; in the evening they sit badly and with cramped muscles in front of the television until it is time to go to bed. They would be very much healthier if they spent the time in the fresh air instead. Those children who are naturally good at sports and are encouraged to take part in them at school will suffer least from such problems (provided their bad posture is corrected rather than reinforced by their teachers). But, as Professor Kraus again points out, some form of physical education is essential for *all* children, whether gifted or not, and it should find a place in educational curricula from primary school to university. When, in addition, life within the family is strained and unhappy, the child is continually living with tension that sooner or later will take its toll.

I know from my own experience what it means to grow up without the advantage of good health. A difficult childhood and many illnesses led me very early in life along a lonely road. Yoga helped me at that time to say Yes to a life that for me was no longer worth living. At first I was in such bad physical condition that I could no longer manage a normal programme of exercises. But, gradually and alone, I learnt first to breathe properly and then grew stronger and conquered my almost permanent feeling of exhaustion. The influence of positive thinking was another step forward. Then I learnt to sit properly, to stand properly and to hold myself properly whatever I was doing. In this way I gradually unburdened my hitherto so easily exhausted body. I learnt to sleep deeply so that it restored and healed me and I could relax easily. Yoga helped me to overcome my limited powers of movement and very gradually I found myself back in a life which now became both precious and full of depth and beauty. Often I thought how wonderful it would be to give everyone the key to such a life in childhood, before it had time to be destroyed.

We must not succumb to the illusion that children are very limited in what they can feel and understand. They have an immense capacity to respond, something which we ourselves must newly discover as we have often lost it in our externally ordered world. It is not, in the first instance, important for the child to understand the full significance of what he is doing.

Once children have come into contact with yoga they have

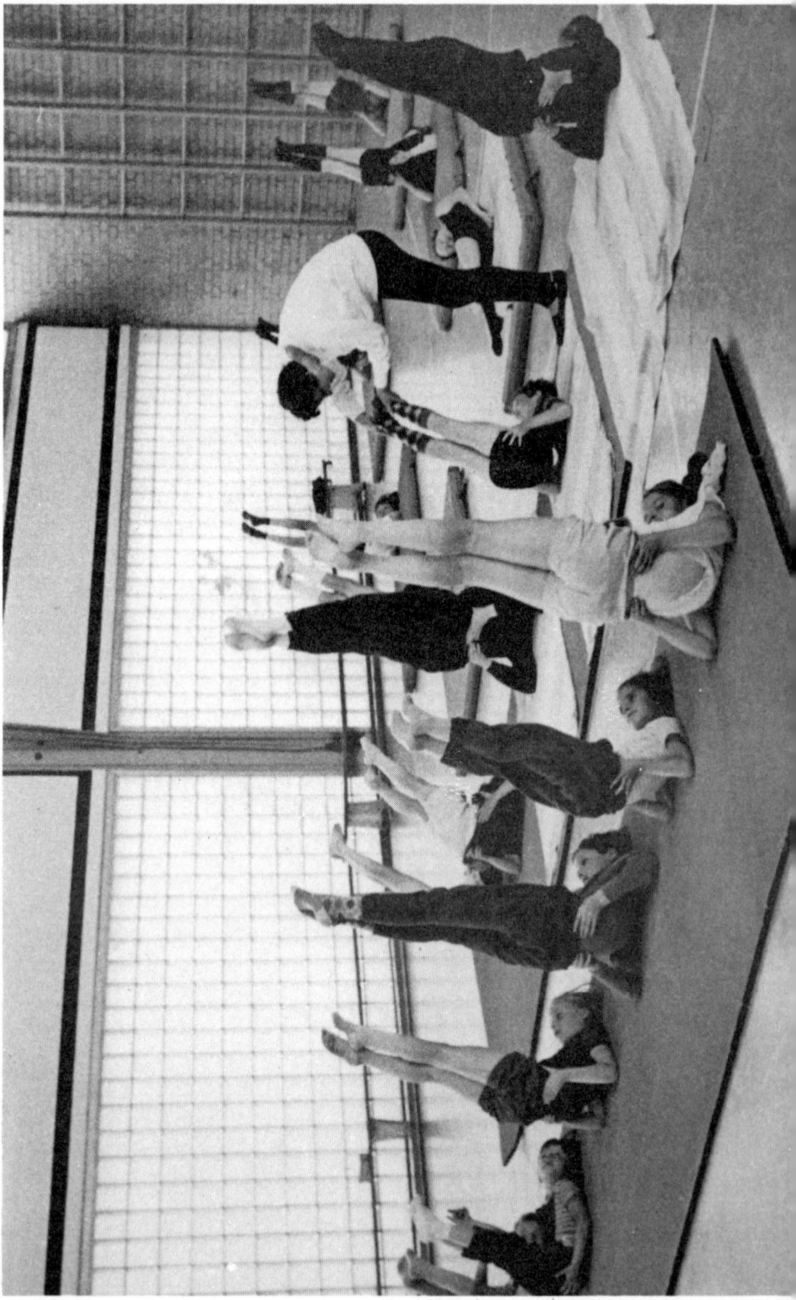

not only a means of keeping healthy, but also (though they may not at first realize it) access to sources of spiritual strength which they will never completely lose, and which in moments of difficulty in later life, can be of enormous importance to them. Yoga gives young people the necessary mental and physical strength for the demands they must meet on their journey through life.

My children's yoga group grew out of these reflections. Very quickly I came to realize that one couldn't assume that children had unlimited strength and suppleness; some of the exercises were at least as difficult for them as for adults. Some children lacked the necessary physical strength, and others, who were tense and restless, found it difficult to relax sufficiently. It also took time for them to correct their faults of posture (some had already developed a hollow back). In the exercises which improved their balance — and these developed not just their physical poise but their psychological stability as well — I could see how, after a while, they began to concentrate hard. Gradually I succeeded in helping even the physically weaker children to become proficient at the relatively advanced exercises.

At first I thought that to spend an hour in absolute quiet and stillness would be too much to ask of children, and that they would stop coming to the classes. But happily the opposite proved to be the case; they came very enthusiastically. One or two of them may have found the first class strange and a little boring but the spirit within the group helped them to overcome the early difficulties. What helps children most is for a parent or elder brother or sister to find the time to spend a few minutes every day doing the exercises with them.

An episode in a yoga lesson

The yoga lesson must be so arranged that it brings the children from restlessness to complete calm. It is fascinating to watch how hard the children work and how afterwards they lie completely relaxed. The end of my first class particularly impressed me. The children were lying on their backs in the savasana position with their eyes closed. Slowly they sat up and I told them they could stand up and go home. But what did they do? After a normal school lesson they would have jumped up and disappeared from the room in the twinkling of an eye; but instead they remained sitting in front of me, calm and reflective. I had to tell them again that the class was finished as they needed quite a long time to re-adjust to the everyday world. Their calm reflectiveness was unforgettable and it showed that it had been possible to lead them back into themselves. An hour spent in this way freed them from all outside tensions and created a quite different atmosphere. The following example is particularly illuminating:

A little boy in the class, who was especially inhibited and often found the lesson difficult, used always to try to avoid doing the exercises with the rest of the class; naturally he made every effort not to be noticed. As the lesson was obviously helping him so little, I decided to try an experiment: very gently I encouraged him to demonstrate to the other children one of the exercises he had just failed to take part in. Very self-consciously he did what I asked him, trying his hardest. The great risk was that the other children might have laughed at him, or that being singled out for attention might have inhibited him still further. But they watched him, quiet and interested, and clapped in acknowledgment. No one talked and the stillness was not broken.

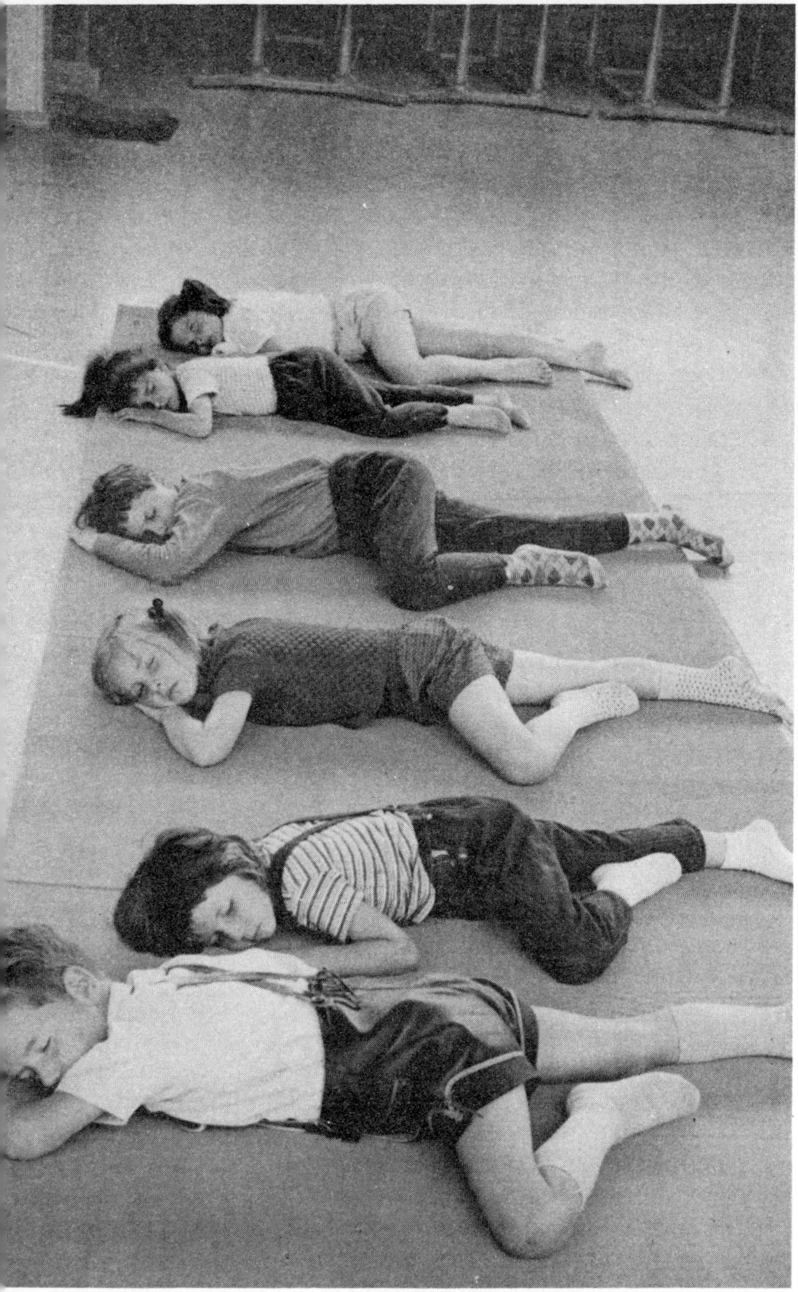

Relaxation during the lesson

Every now and again I begin the class by telling an Indian fairy story. This puts the children at their ease; they are still and attentive and follow every word with rapt attention. I am certain that they interpret in their own way the deep and mysterious meaning which is hidden in all fairy stories. I should like to tell one of the stories here as it has something very important to say to us about the meaning of human happiness. It is the Indian fairy tale about the tree that granted every wish:

'A young man had set his heart on finding the tree which would make every wish come true. To this end he wandered hither and thither through the dense primeval forest of the Himalayas. After he had searched for a long time he found the tree and, persuaded that his troubles were at an end, he gazed at it in wonder.

"How marvellous it would be to possess a sack full of gold", thought the young man. And at that moment heaps of glittering gold appeared before his astonished eyes. Speechless with happiness he wished for a chest of jewels. And this too lay at his feet scarcely before his wish was complete. "I'll have a palace of pure gold", he cried, and one appeared before him in all its glistening splendour. Hungry and tired after his long walk, he wished for something to eat; and without delay a richly laid table appeared. He ate and ate until he was so full he couldn't eat any more. "A beautiful soft bed to lie down on", he requested next. And a pure gold one stood ready at his feet. As he lay down it suddenly occurred to him that he was in the middle of a dark forest. "What if a tiger should come and eat me up?" he thought. Scarcely had the thought flitted through his head, when really and truly a tiger appeared, fell on him and ate him up.

The human heart is like the tree. It grants both the good and the evil wishes'.

How marvellously this story portrays the power of wishes; and it should warn us to treat them with circumspection and to recognize that thought has similar powers. Children know this already: perhaps they receive things they secretly longed for, or things have gone wrong when they knew they would. Haven't we all experienced this?

Children and their environment

The child's environment can have an important bearing on his whole life. I remember very clearly the time when I worked at an orphanage and there, among the infants and young children, were illegitimate children taken into care and offered for adoption. Although they were not living with their parents they were well looked-after and received every care and attention. And yet there was something missing: the loving regard of someone who cared for each of them individually and provided the warmth and support necessary for their happiness.

Another unforgettable time was shortly before the end of the war, when many people had fled, bringing their few remaining possessions with them. My home-town was filled with refugees and it was an everyday occurrence to see, after an air-raid, lost and fleeing children roaming through the streets. They were quite silent and, like everyone else, hungry. They looked uncared for and stared out of huge vacant eyes. They rarely begged for bread because they had already learnt that people no longer had any to give, and often with aching heart I saw a child such as this, its grubby fingers in its mouth.

Today, our main concern is with improving living standards, and even mothers with several children continue to go out to work so as to help pay for the better, but more expensive flat, the car or the television. Amidst so much prosperity the children's interests take second place.

Children will therefore always be dependent on adults: on the living conditions created for them, and on their ideas of what is good and bad; it is the adult who decides when they go to bed, what they eat and how they should be dressed. If children are to be true to their own personalities, it is essential that adults consider their real interests, and instead of stifling their attempts at independence, help them towards it.

A correct diet is basic to children's health. The diet should be healthy and nutritious, consisting of food that retains all its natural ingredients. Highly-seasoned, over-cooked and adulterated foods lack the nutrients essential for young and growing bodies; what children need above all is vitamins not in concen-

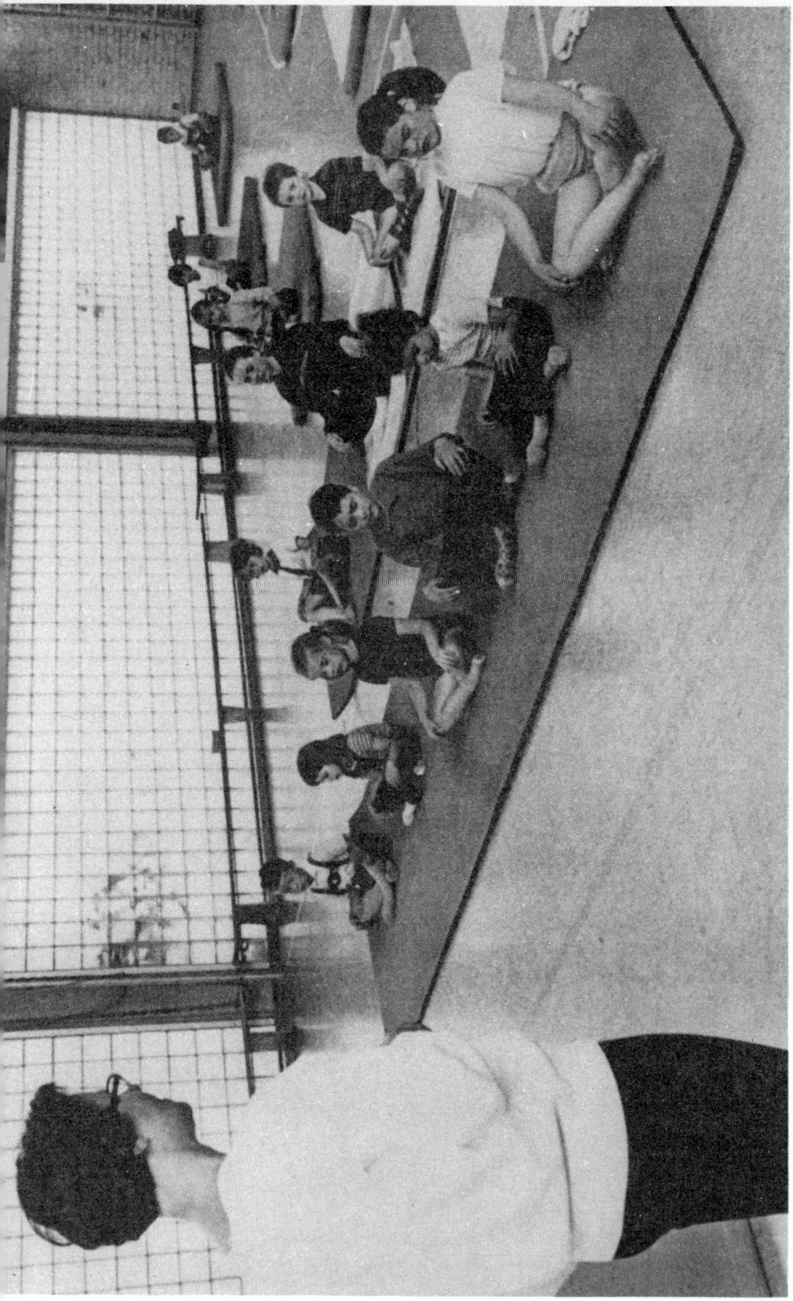

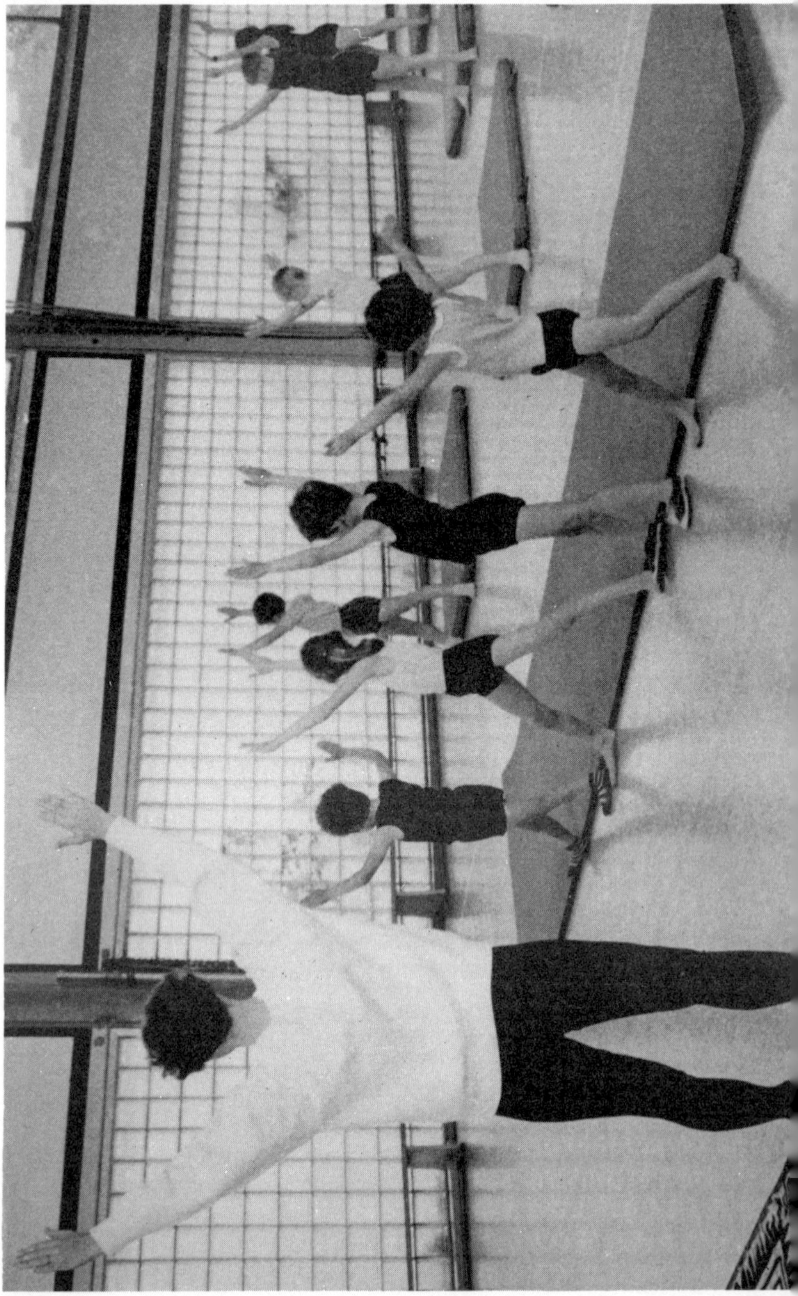

trated form but as they are found in natural foods. Processed convenience foods have none of the nutritional value of meals made from fresh ingredients; milk, fruit, vegetables, wholewheat and salad which are essential for the health of growing children.

Unfortunately our food today includes cakes, biscuits, chocolate and ice-cream, sweet things eaten while watching television, and instead of home-made wholemeal bread, sweets eaten on the way to school and in the morning break; there is the all too popular practice of giving children sweets and biscuits in bed. Only ignorance makes it possible for so many people to succumb so unreservedly to a taste that slowly but surely will make them ill.

Doctors and nutrition experts are agreed on the harmful effects of eating white sugar and refined flour. As a result of food processing white sugars and flours are turned into completely chemical products, robbed of their natural ingredients. In order to function normally the metabolism requires vitamins, minerals and trace elements that are found in sweet fruit, wholewheat and sugarbeet, but which are no longer present in refined products. Where these are missing, the body is forced to draw on its own resources with the result that the metabolism is thrown off balance. Refined sugar and flour are responsible, therefore, not only for tooth decay but perhaps even for cancer as well as other diseases of the 'civilized' world.

It is little wonder therefore that the children we 'delight' with sweet things, fail to thrive on them. Nor is it surprising that children who are continually given chocolate are nervous and irritable and ask for it more and more often as their sense of taste deteriorates and their natural physical requirements are thrown off balance. The way to help children is in not allowing them to become addicted to unhealthy eating habits in the first place. It is all too easy to leave a child to its own devices but adults should bear the ultimate responsibility and use their love and judgment in the child's best interests. However beneficial, yoga can be of little use if children continue in a way of life that is so prejudicial to their health and well-being.

In the same way that children need food for their bodies they need adults' love and understanding for their souls. How important it is to do justice to children's spiritual needs and to realize that so-called temper tantrums stem from genuine psychological problems; for these are their way of protesting

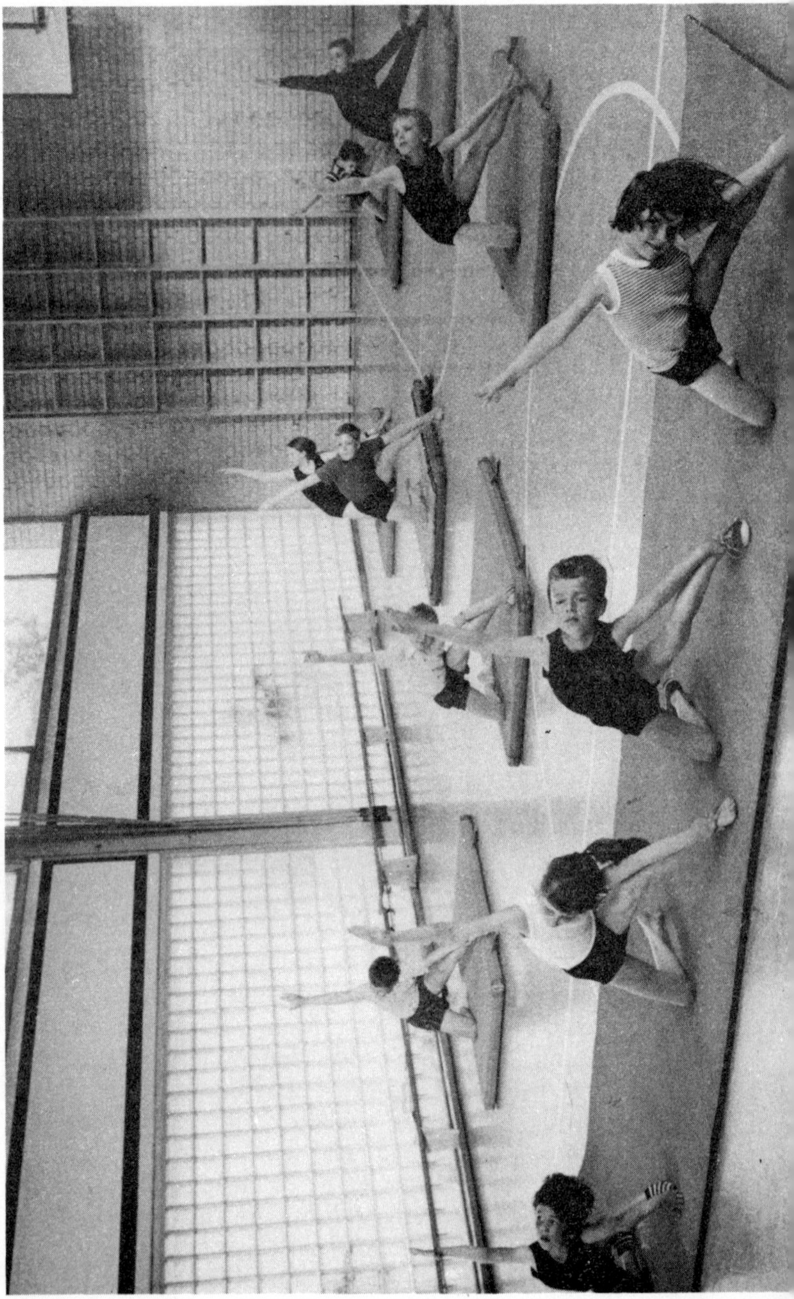

against a situation that is unbearable to them. Children who are psychologically repressed cannot develop into people who are happy and healthy and who whole-heartedly accept life. Psychological problems are often the cause of physical illnesses which may only appear at a later stage. But children will be mentally and physically strong if they experience encouragement and feel that they are surrounded by the protective wall of a caring relationship; not one which oppresses them but one which allows them to grow up in the greatest possible freedom.

We should try to ensure that children are psychologically equipped to cope with life's demands and those which we ourselves make of them. We can help children to find their own way by patiently allowing them time and an absence of pressure so that they can turn back and draw on their own limitless human resources. Here I should like to recount a personal experience which demonstrates vividly that it is not always the most expensive toys which give children the greatest pleasure.

In a Swiss mountain village, a truly lonely spot, I watched a little boy of about five years old who was playing in front of his parents' house. The farmers in this tiny village worked hard and lived simply. He was plainly and sensibly dressed and was playing with a couple of stones and the sand on the path. In one hand he held a branch, just picked from a nearby tree. As I crossed the road, he came over to me, and stretching out his arm, barred my way. With eyes sparkling with life, he looked me up and down and asked 'What's your name?' After I had told him and he had appraised me still further, he held out his right hand and said: 'Look what a good stick I've got!' With these words his face lit up for it was for him at that moment the most beautiful thing he possessed. He asked me if I would like one too and was convinced that there could be no more valuable present than a branch like his. Very carefully he picked one for me and peeled off the leaves. As he handed it to me, I looked into two shining eyes.

This child lived close to nature, was surrounded by beauty and freedom and experienced them to their depths. Nothing troubled him, no march of time, and he played to the accompaniment of the rustling of the leaves in the trees, the cowbells and the sound of the wind in the snow-covered mountains. When this child went to bed he could look through his tiny window at a star-filled sky infinite in its breadth and depth.

We who live in an urban society are estranged from nature and fail to find the necessary relaxation and harmony that its stillness and beauty bring.

It is precisely here that yoga can help for it restores the lost harmony between body, mind and spirit and shows us the road that leads back to ourselves and to nature. We shall want to learn once again to listen to the silence which can say far more to us than the ever-present background noise. Deep union with nature brings us all those things — above all the gift of real health — which in the civilized world are so obviously absent.

Children are much closer to the natural and the divine, for adults have reasoned away those things which are still real to children though part of 'another world'. It is not children who so often give something to adults, from whom adults can learn? How beautifully the words of Bô yin Râ express this:

> Have you ever seen a child that has built a sand castle
> and claps his hands when his work is complete?
> Here you have found your master, you who strive after happiness . . . .
> Here is someone who has found happiness.
> Like the child, do not seek to be happy, for your search will bring only needless suffering and pain.

On the same theme Vivekanada writes: 'Never say "mine". As soon as we say "this is mine" then misery has us in its clutches. Don't say even to yourself, in your thoughts, "this is my child". Have the child but don't call it "mine" for once you do your life will be filled with sorrow'. If we take these words to heart then we shall also understand the poet Kahlil Gibran:

> Your children are not your children.
> They are the sons and daughters of
> Life's longing for itself.
> They come through you but not from you,
> And though they are with you yet they
> belong not to you.
> You may give them your love but not
> your thoughts,

For they have their own thoughts.
You may house their bodies but not
their souls,
For their souls dwell in the house of
tomorrow, which you cannot visit, not
even in your dreams.
You may strive to be like them, but seek
not to make them like you.
For life goes not backward nor tarries
with yesterday.
You are the bows from which your children
as living arrows are sent forth.
. . .
Let your bending in the archer's hand be for gladness;

(Kahlil Gibran, *The Prophet*).

Calm — source of strength

Our greatest source of strength is the peace within us. A person who meets life with serenity and composure handles difficulties differently from someone who has lost his inner tranquility. Without this inner peace we are like a ball in the hands of fate. Someone who is not at peace with himself will try also to avoid external silence, and it is understandable that in the stillness of the forests people carry transistor radios, and that swimming pools and camping sites, despite the beauty of nature all around them, are places of noise and confusion. For to many people the stillness and peace of nature are literally unbearable and they therefore drive it away.

Naturally people's inner uneasiness is at its greatest when outside noise suddenly ceases. Silence which we should experience with gratitude becomes a source of torment. So we shouldn't wonder when the peace which should fall with night-time is disturbed, and sleep, instead of bringing a longed-for relief, is troubled. We have broken away from nature and destroyed the harmony, the balance between rest and activity; we have turned the nights into days. A good cup of coffee dispels the feeling of tiredness; when we turn the knob of the television, the sound of welcome conversation breaks in on us; after an exhausting day we need something to help us relax and there is an enormous variety of such distractions. The technical means we have created to enrich our lives are truly fantastic. How differently our ancestors, for example, spent their evenings. After a long and hard day's work they would sit in front of the house on an old bench and listen to the rustling of the leaves in the trees. They lived in closest harmony with nature, put their trust in her creative strength and felt themselves one with her.

Today's world is far removed from this ancient way of life, for technical progress and greater prosperity do not afford the feeling of inner accord and belonging that we need to live in perfect harmony. We ourselves know how gratifying we find the calm and tranquillity that some people radiate. If a mother feeds her baby when she herself is worried and distracted, he doesn't go peacefully to sleep, he cries; and young children are

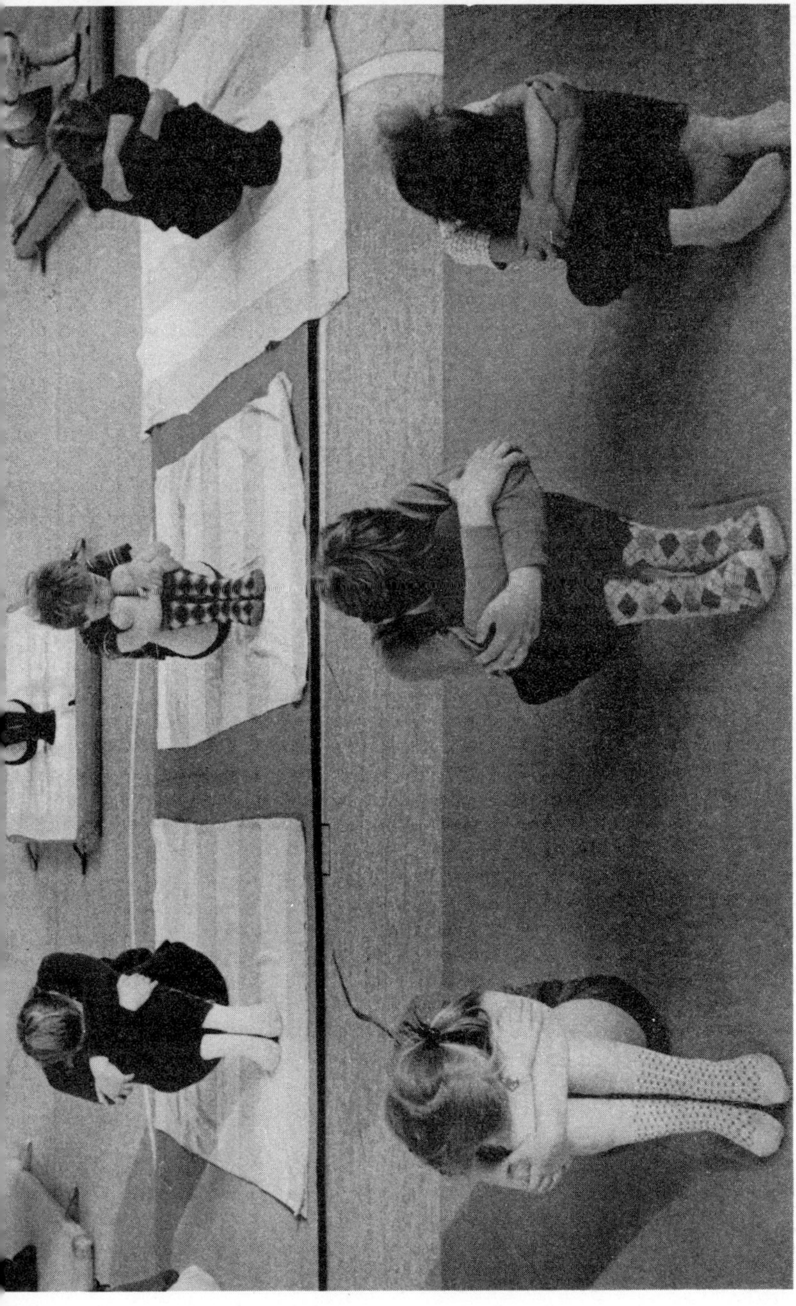

similarly vulnerable to the moods and emotions of their parents. We should try to ensure that our children grow up surrounded by peace and contentment and that they do not gradually lose their own natural feeling of tranquillity. Children need a quiet and peaceful environment and no television programme (no matter how good) is an adequate substitute.

Not fearing silence or loneliness, we should use each undisturbed moment that the day may send us, to find peace within ourselves and oneness with the whole of creation. Selvarajan Yesudian, a wise teacher, once said to his pupil: 'You cry and call on God whom you cannot see. Open your eyes and perceive God in the beauty of the flowers, in the scent of the rose, in the friendly light of the stars, in the majesty of the mountains, in the wild torrents of the streams, in death, and in the birth of each child'.

Let us once again find a place for quietude in our lives. Let us be grateful that night brings us new strength for the day ahead and, rather than seeking to shorten these hours, let us use them to the full. Anxiety, fear and despair will have no place in us, and we shall draw on mysterious sources of power and enjoy life.

The importance of correct breathing

With the first breath life begins. Human beings can live for about four weeks without solid food and survive a few days without liquids. But unless we breathe, life ceases immediately. In inverse order man needs first food, then liquids but most important of all, breathing. It is not food but breathing 'which keeps body and soul together'. 'For breath is life' says an old Sanskrit proverb, 'and when you breathe well, you will live long'. But to be able to breathe well, we must breathe correctly: through the nose. For breathing is not just a matter of inhaling and exhaling air; it affects our whole physical and mental well-being. Look how miserable we feel when a really heavy cold and a blocked-up nose prevents us from breathing properly.

Mouth-breathing is inadequate for it does not replace the vital energy which streams into the body when we breathe through the nose and which the yogis call 'prana'. And nose-breathing has another function: that of protecting us from infections carried into the body by bacilli. We shouldn't be surprised if we succumb to infectious diseases when we breathe through our mouths. Yet another function of the nose is to filter out the dust particles and other foreign bodies and to warm the cold air that we breathe in. We know that the mouth has quite other functions to perform and can never completely take over the work of the nose. Although nature in her wisdom has made it possible for us to breathe through our mouths when we really have to, if we want to resist infections and remain healthy we must learn to breathe through our noses.

Children who are fearful or have an inferiority complex often hunch their shoulders and thus prevent the full expansion of their lungs. Children who are encouraged to breathe properly lose this feeling of fear, become more self-confident and less susceptible to colds and other diseases.

It is important to ensure that from their earliest years children breathe through their noses. They will not only be stronger and healthier, more balanced and at peace with themselves, but will

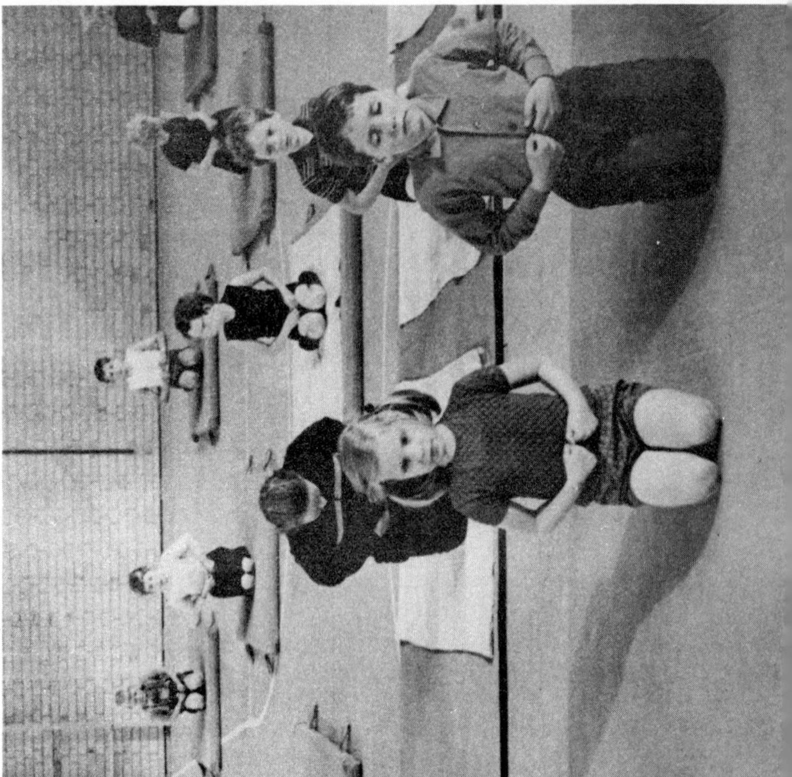

have in addition a greater potential for spiritual development.

We should be careful only to practise 'full-breathing' — like all hatha-yoga exercises — on an empty stomach and only to begin when we are completely relaxed (through *savasana*).

'Full-breathing' consists of three consecutive and inter-related stages:

1. the so-called abdominal or diaphragm breathing
2. middle breathing
3. upper breathing.

Before attempting 'full-breathing' you should master the individual stages.

Control of abdominal or diaphragm breathing:

Sit cross-legged (or lie on your back) with your hands on your abdomen (not your stomach) and breathe in gently, let your diaphragm expand. Breathing out slowly, let your diaphragm fall. Repeat twice.

Control of middle breathing:

Sit cross-legged with your hands on either side of your chest. Feel how your chest expands as you breathe in and contracts as you slowly breathe out. Repeat twice.

Control of upper breathing:

Sit crosslegged with your hands on your collar bone. As you breathe in feel the lifting of your chest and collar bone when the upper part of your lungs fills with air, and how they sink back again as you breathe out.

Exercise in 'full-breathing'

Sitting cross-legged, put your hands on your knees, close your eyes and work through all the three breathing stages. Each stage should follow naturally on the last without a break. Breathe gently but deeply, never jerkily or straining, and let this way of breathing become completely automatic. Begin with abdominal breathing, followed by middle breathing and then upper breathing. Breathe out in the same sequence, letting the diaphragm sink first, then emptying the middle part of the lungs and lastly the upper part. Each stage should flow into the next, naturally and without effort, like the gentle movement of waves.

'Full-breathing' is most effective either half an hour before a meal or at the beginning of a hatha-yoga session. It should never be practised unless you are fully relaxed and initially not for longer than a minute. After a week you can increase the time to three minutes and at the very most to five minutes.

'Full-breathing' is the basis of all yoga breathing exercises and should be mastered before you proceed to the more advanced stages.

Here I should like to explain another breathing exercise which is both easy to perform and immensely beneficial:

AGNISARA DHAUTI

Sit on your heels (or lie on your back) with your hands on your abdomen (not your stomach). First breathe out, pulling in your abdomen as you do so. Then breathe in sharply, expanding the abdominal wall. Breathing out again, let your abdominal wall sink and pull in the abdomen once again. Repeat twenty times in quick succession but make sure you don't breathe deeply; take only shallow breaths. This exercise cleanses the blood, massages the abdominal organs and helps to prevent constipation, a sluggish liver and disorders of the pancreas.

PART TWO

Exercises and instructions

When doing all these exercises it is important not to strain yourself and not to attempt too much at a time. It is advisable to work under the supervision (if possible medical) of an expert at least until you are sure that you are doing the exercises correctly and not harming yourself.

Never exercise on a full stomach; never rush or hurry but always begin and end each session with the rest position (savasana). Never continue too long: three-quarters of an hour (or at the most an hour) including rest pauses is enough.

Bear in mind that each exercise is followed by a reaction which you cannot prevent taking place. Don't play with powers you don't understand.

Section A (simple exercises):

Section A consists of exercises which you can build into your daily exercise programme.

Section B (intermediate exercises):

The exercises in Section B are more difficult; do them with caution, don't strain yourself, be patient.

Section C (advanced exercises):

These exercises should only be included in your programme when you have mastered those in section B and can perform them with ease.

Twisting exercises:

Twisting exercises should also be done with caution. Their simplicity is deceptive. Include only one twisting exercise in each session.

Breathing control

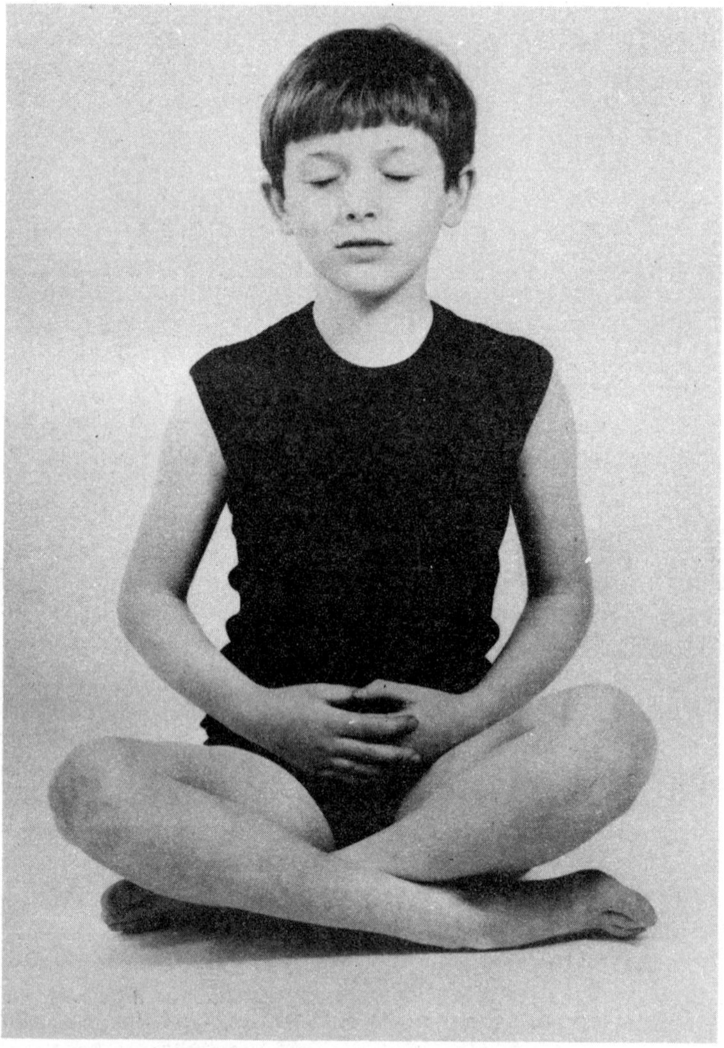

Control of abdominal or diaphragm breathing

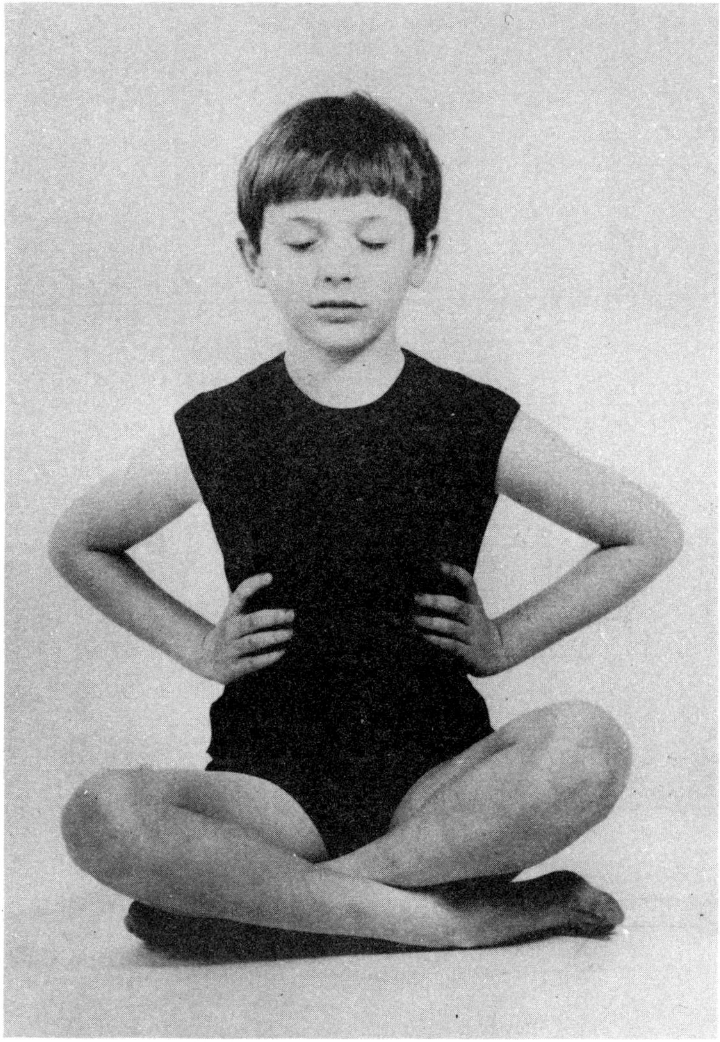

Control of middle breathing

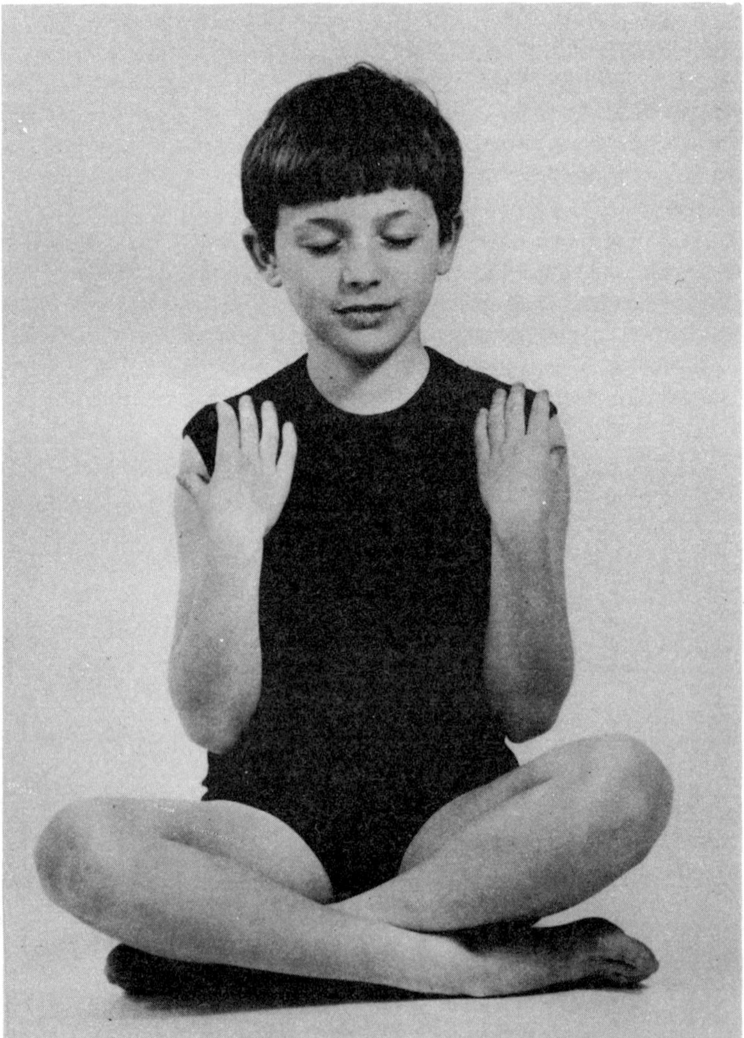

Control of upper breathing

Breathing exercises

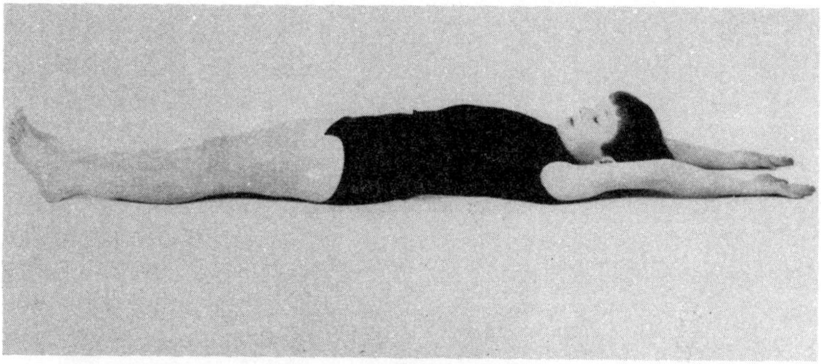

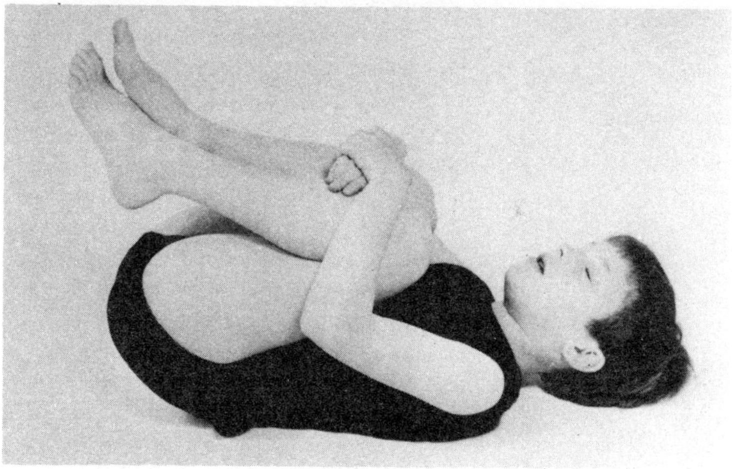

HA-breathing

Lie on your back. Breathing in deeply, stretch your arms out on the floor behind your head. Breathe out quickly and bend your legs up against your chest, hugging both knees. After about ten seconds lower your legs to the floor. Breathing in, lift your arms over your head and, continuing to breathe slowly through your nose, lay them to rest at your sides. Repeat twice. (Cleanses the abdominal organs; improves circulation.)

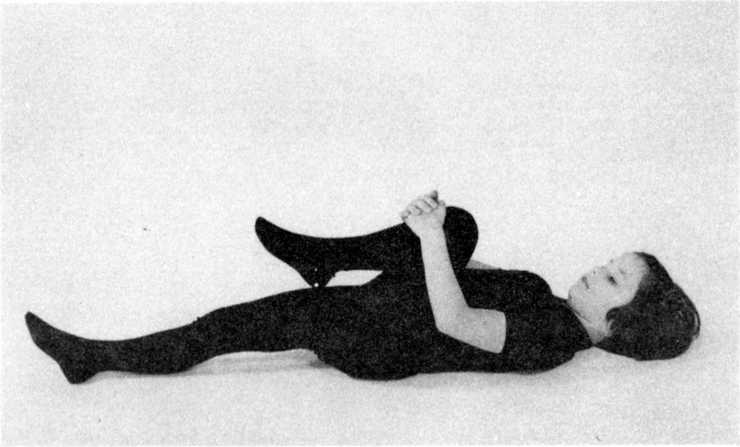

ARDHA-HA-breathing

Lie on your back and breathing in deeply lay your arms on the floor stretched out behind your head. Breathing out quickly through your mouth, hug your right knee. After about ten seconds lower your right leg to the floor and while breathing in stretch out your arms again on the floor behind your head. Breathing out quickly through your mouth, hug your left knee and after about ten seconds lower your left leg to the floor. Breathing in, raise both arms and breathing out slowly lay them to rest at either side. Repeat twice.
(Cleanses the abdominal organs; improves circulation.)

Rest positions

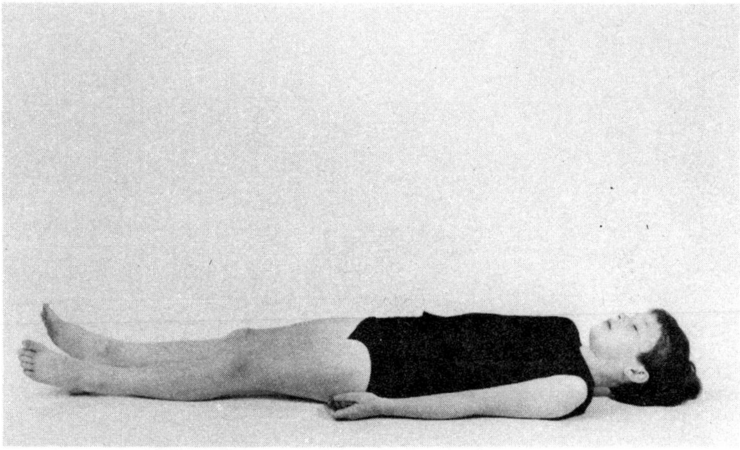

SAVASANA

Lie on your back, your arms by your sides. Breathe peacefully and deeply, as slowly as you can without straining. Relax all the muscles of your body, concentrating on each one as you do so. Your body should be so relaxed that you no longer feel it. Don't let your mind wander but collect all your distracting thoughts together and then forget them so you experience only the deepest peace.
(Calms the nerves; relaxes the muscles; strengthens the heart; improves circulation.)

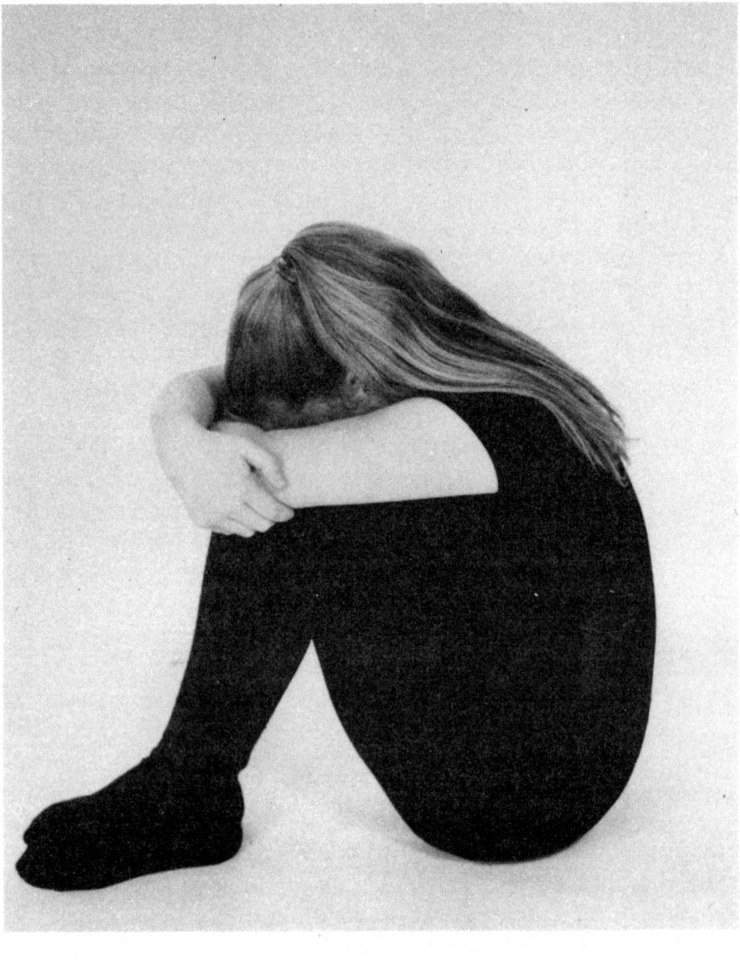

Rest position

Sit with your knees drawn up to your chin. Hug your knees and rest your forehead on them.

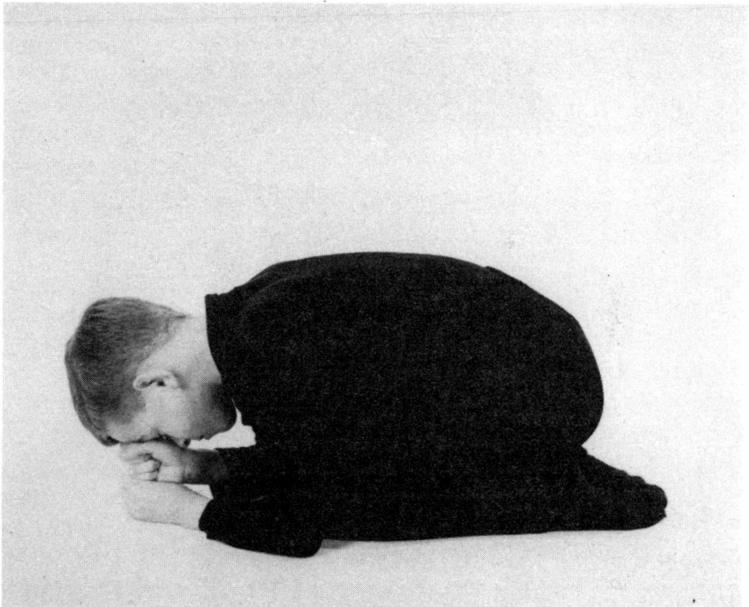

Rest position

Sit on your heels, bend right forward and rest your forehead on your hands. Your fists should be lightly clenched and placed one on top of the other.

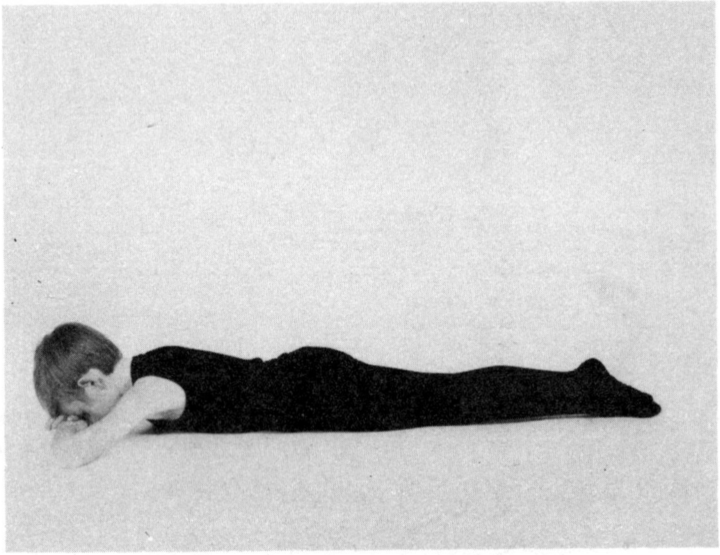

Rest position

Lie face down on the floor, your forehead resting on your hands.

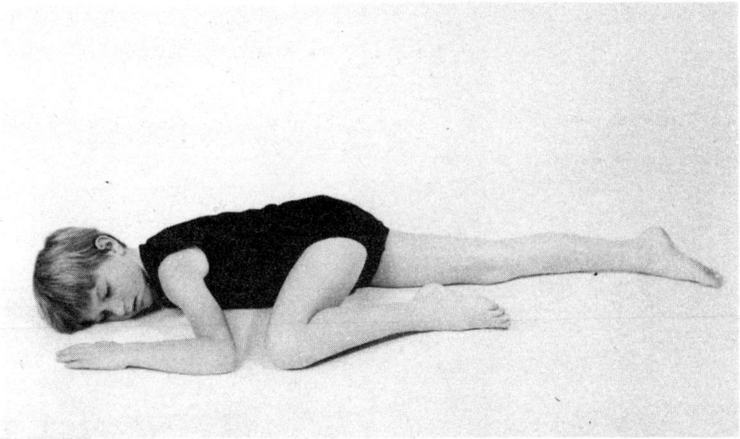

Lie on your stomach, your right leg straight, your right arm resting by your side. Lay your head on your right ear and keep your left leg and arm bent. After about a minute, reverse the position.
(Calms the nervous system: reduces insomnia.)

This is also an ideal sleeping position. I have encountered some evidence to suggest that there is a correlation between children's sleeping positions and their ability to learn to read. This is not surprising for the way a child sleeps affects the working of his entire nervous system. Children who instinctively sleep in the position shown on this page seem to have relatively few reading difficulties, whereas children who do not have a fixed sleeping position seem to be generally unco-ordinated (in my experience anyway — you can observe this in the way they run, jump or write) and to have corresponding difficulties in learning to read.

Starting positions

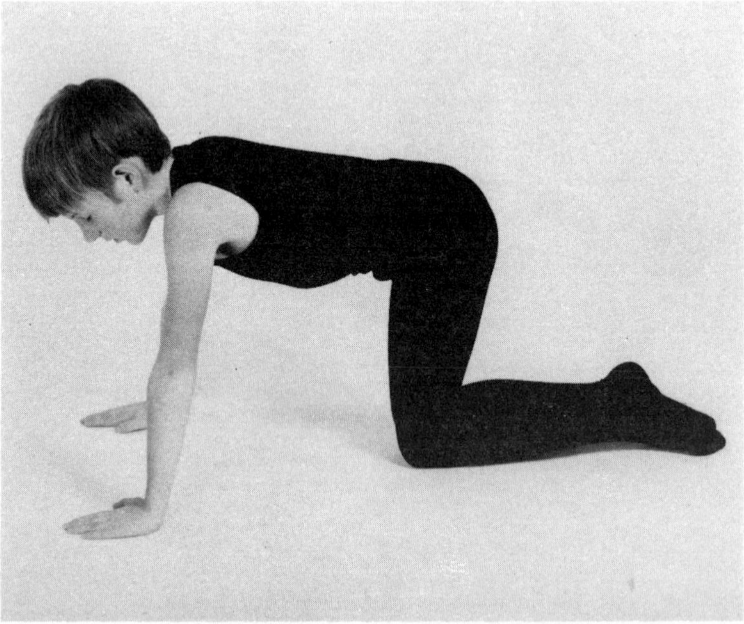

Starting position: on all fours

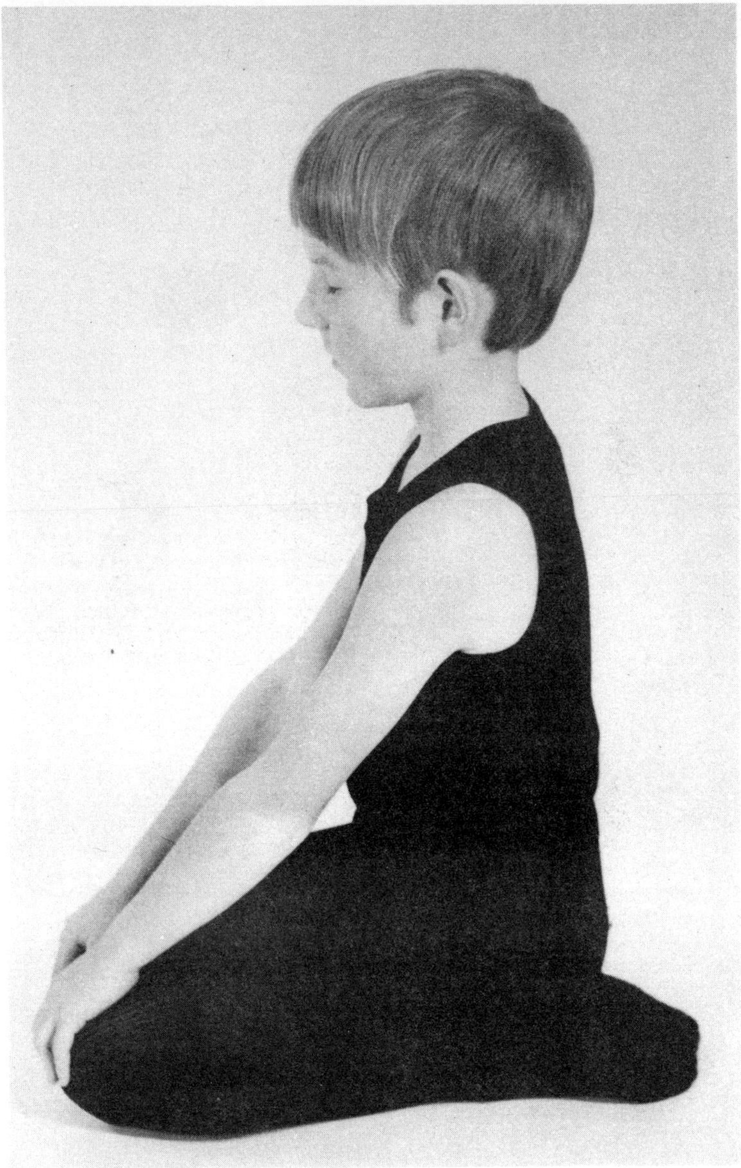

Starting position: sitting on your heels

Sit on your heels so the tops of your feet are flat on the floor and your toes stretched out behind you.

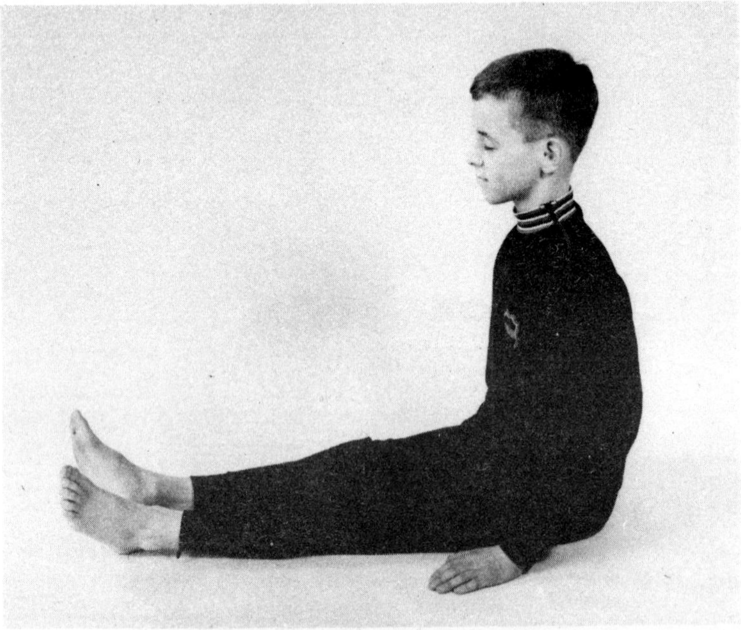

Starting position: sitting with your legs stretched out in front

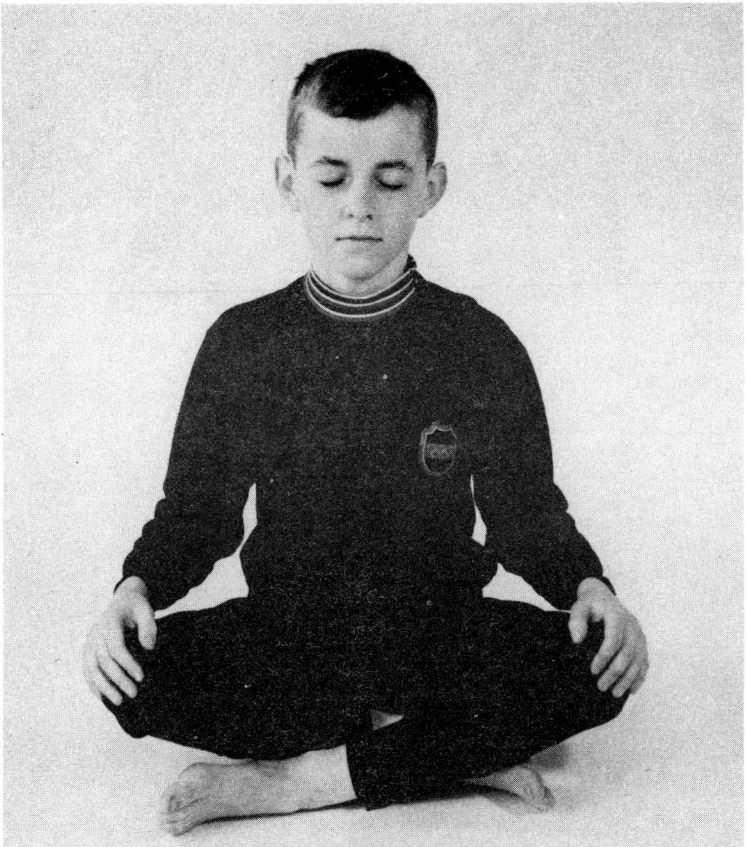

Starting position: cross-legged or tailor squat

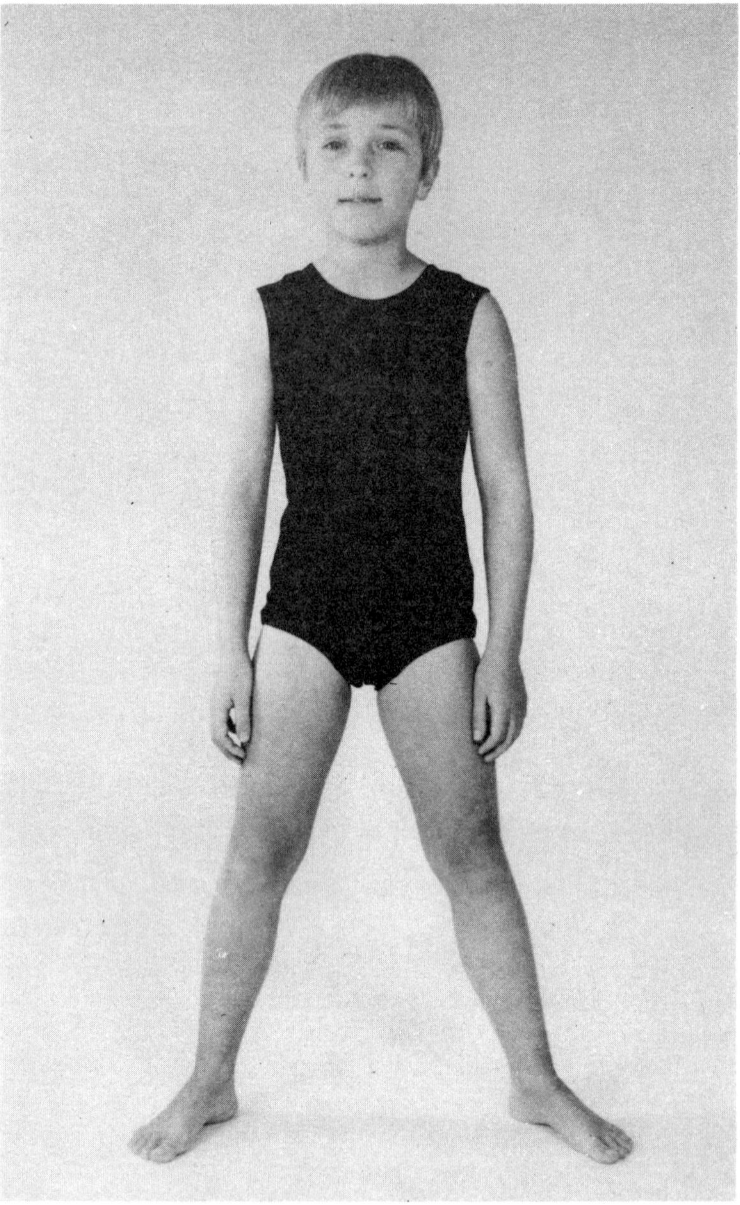

Starting position: straddle-position

Section A exercises

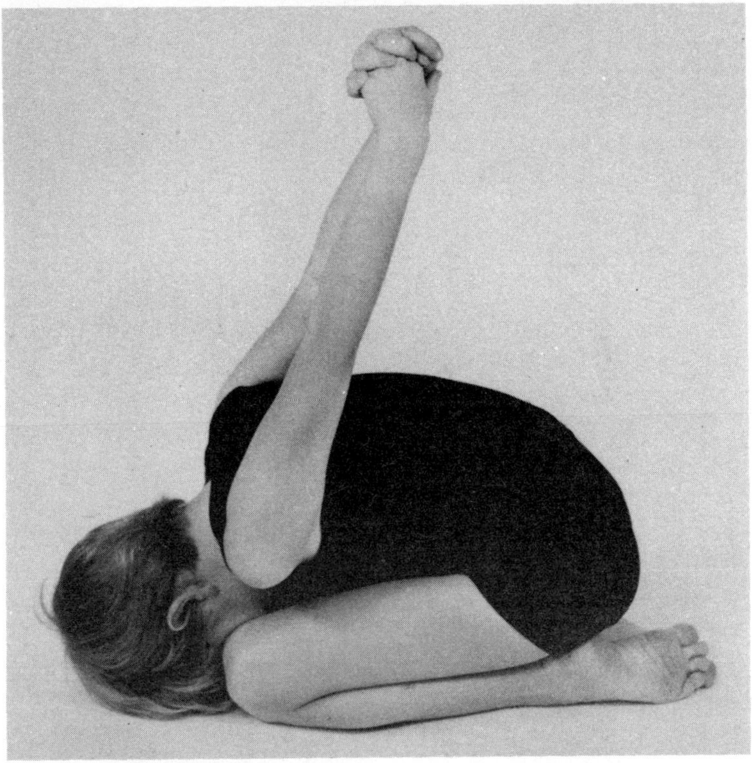

YOGA-MUDRA variation

Sit on your heels and breathe in deeply. Hold your arms behind your back, your hands clasped or folded together. Breathing out, bend forward until your forehead touches the floor and stretch your arms up behind you. Hold the position for about ten seconds without breathing. Then, breathing in, sit up, unclasp your hands and rest them on your knee. Breathe peacefully. After a breathing pause, repeat the exercise twice. Then rest, bent forward supporting your forehead on your fists which should be lightly clenched, one placed on top of the other.

(Strengthens the back muscles, collar bone and shoulder blades; deepens breathing.)

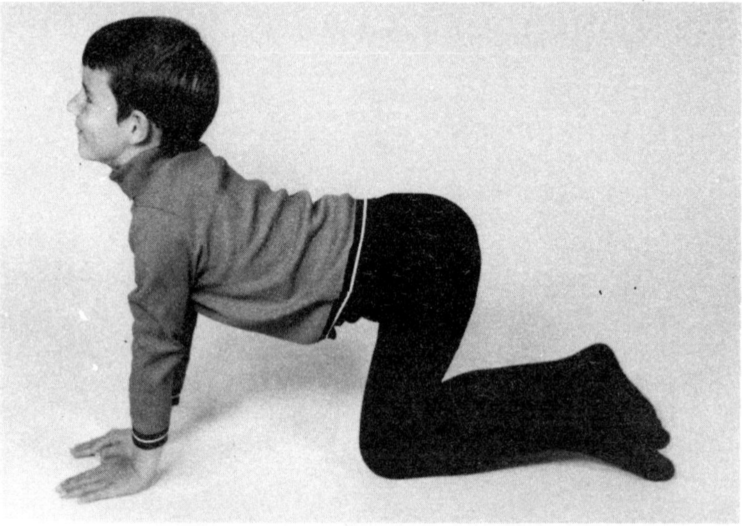

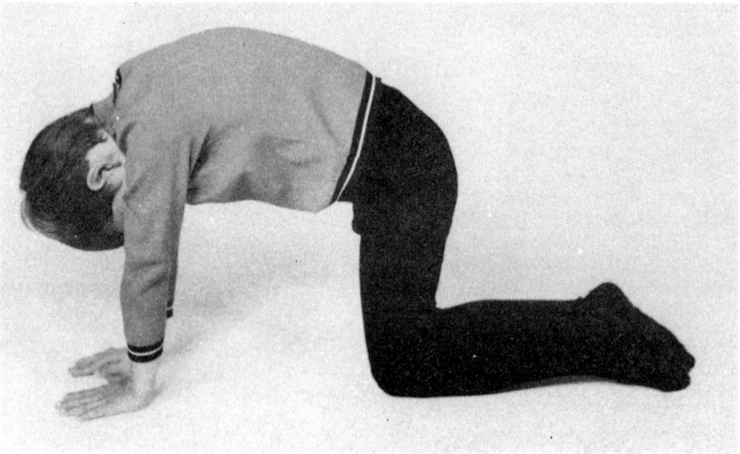

Adopt the 'all-fours' position (your hands and knees on the floor). Breathing in, lower the small of your back simultaneously raising your head. Breathing out, pull in your abdomen, raise the small of your back and at the same time lower your head. Repeat twice then sit on your heels and bend forward, resting your head on your fists.

(Strengthens the spine and stomach muscles.)

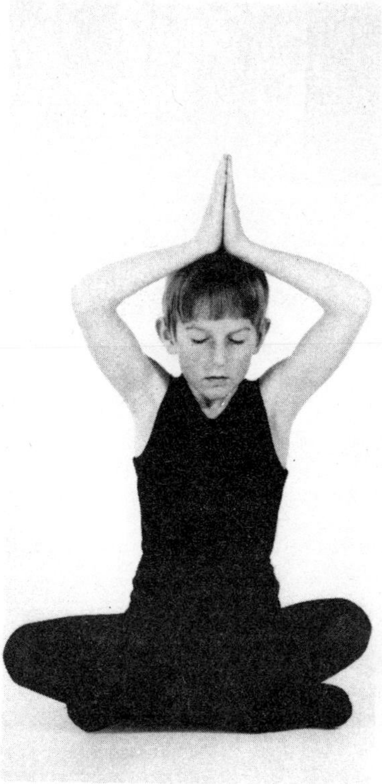

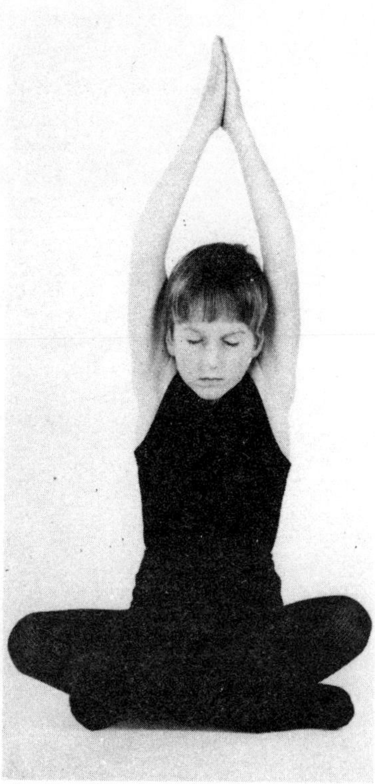

PARVATASANA (*mountain position*)

Sit either cross-legged or on your heels. Breathe in, raise your arms and hold them directly over your head, your elbows bent and your palms together. Hold your breath, expand your abdominal wall and stretch your arms high above your head. Breathe out, lower your arms and lay your hands on your knee. Repeat twice and then rest on your back (savasana).

(Develops will-power and resistance.)

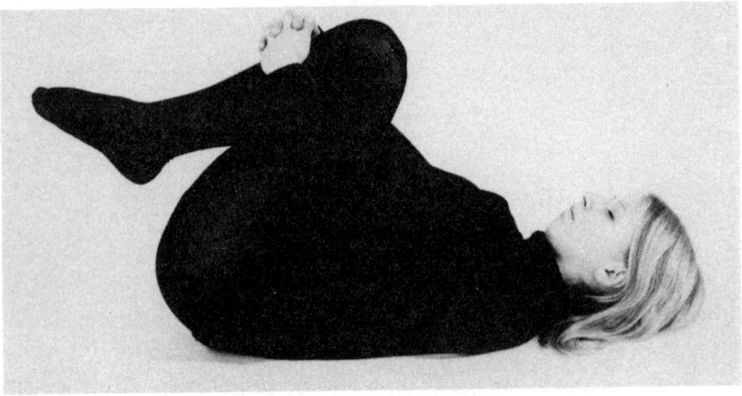

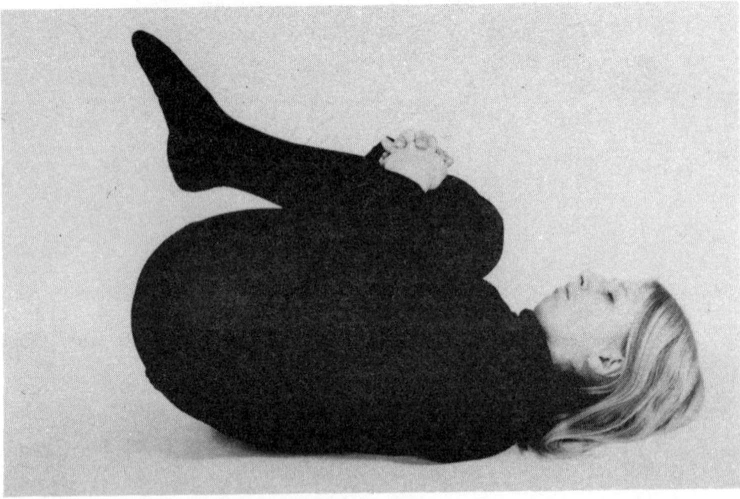

PAVANAMUKTASANA

Lie on your back with your legs drawn up to your chest and your arms encircling both knees. Breathe in deeply. As you breathe out, hug your knees more tightly and pull them closer to your body. Relax your arms again and breathe in. Breathing out, hug your knees more tightly and pull them closer to your body again. Repeat twice and then rest on your back (savasana).

(Tones up all inner organs.)

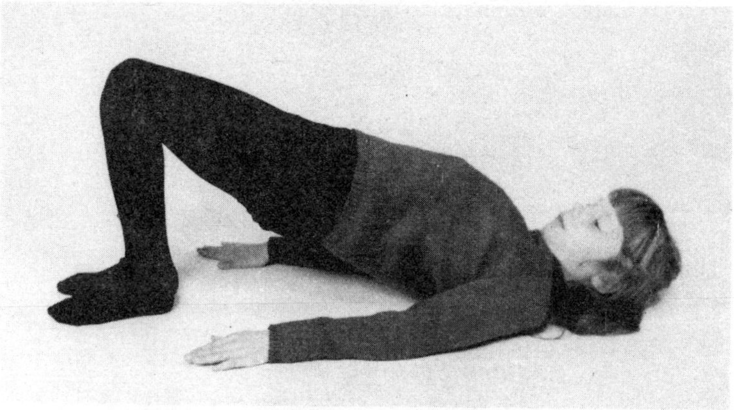

Lie on your back, your arms resting by your side and your palms facing downwards. Your knees should be bent and your feet flat on the floor near your body. Breathing in, gradually raise your back and pelvis off the floor. Breathing out, slowly lower first your shoulders, then your back and lastly your pelvis. Repeat twice, then rest on your back (savasana).

(Counteracts back-ache and stiffness.)

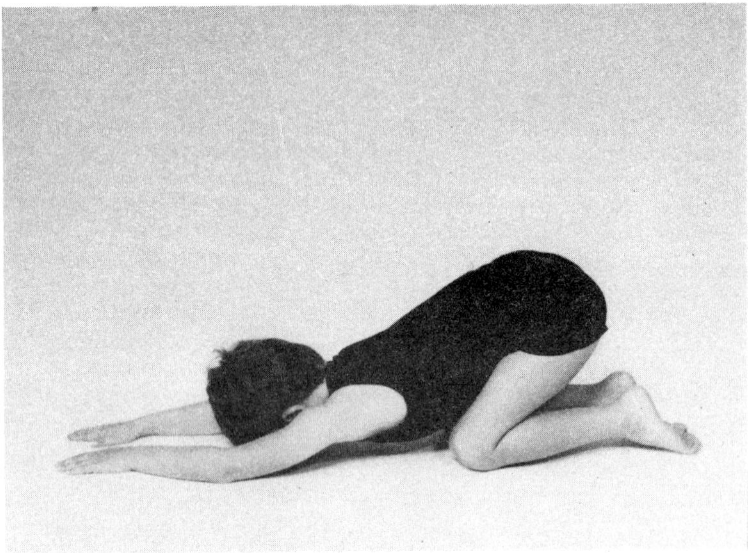

Sit on your heels with your hands on the floor in front of your knees. Then push your arms along the floor until your body is stretched out, your arms taking the weight. Slowly sit back on your heels and rest your hands on your knees. Take a breathing pause then repeat the exercise twice. Rest bent forward supporting your forehead on your fists.

(Strengthens and relaxes a tired back.)

(*See page 56*)

Stand with your feet slightly apart giving yourself plenty of space to move. Breathe in and raise your arms until they are at right-angles to your body. Then breathe out, relax and bend over until your finger tips are touching the floor. Breathe in and stand up straight with your arms outstretched. Then, breathing out slowly, lower your arms. Breathing in, raise your arms and twist your body from the waist upwards to the right. Breathe out, relax and bend over to the right until your finger tips are touching the floor. Breathing in, stand up straight and breathing out, lower your arms. Do the same thing bending to the left. Then rest on your back (savasana).

(Strengthens the abdominal and back muscles.)

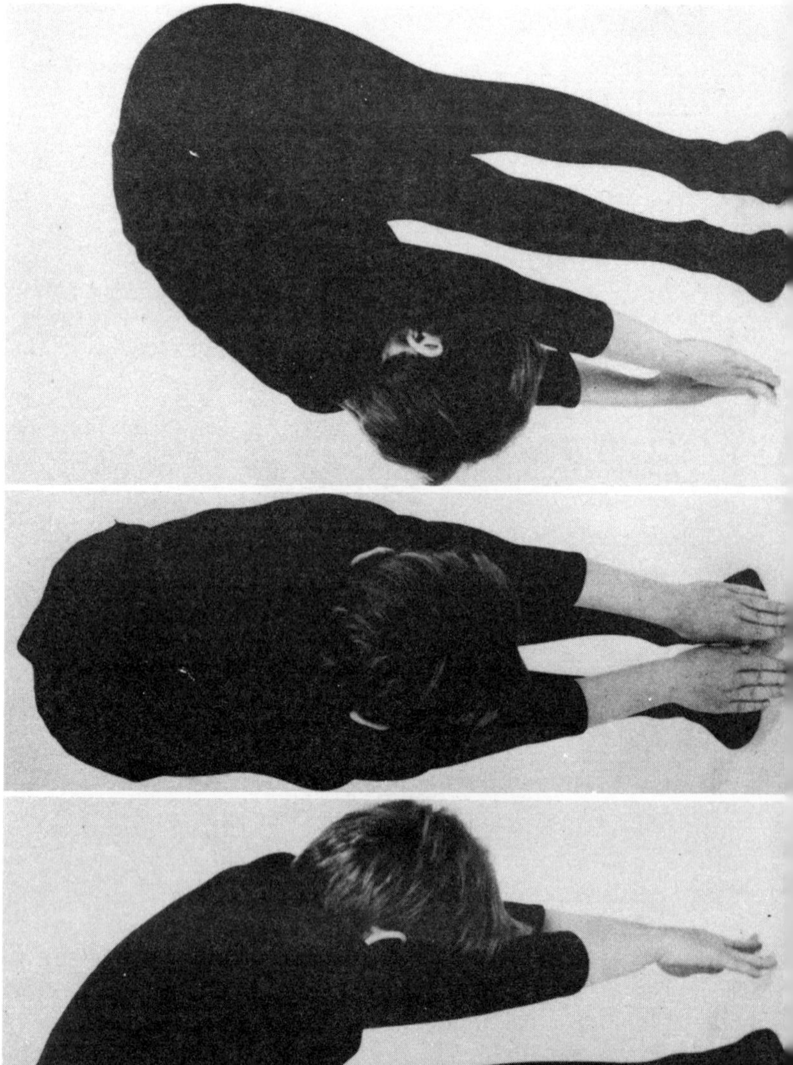

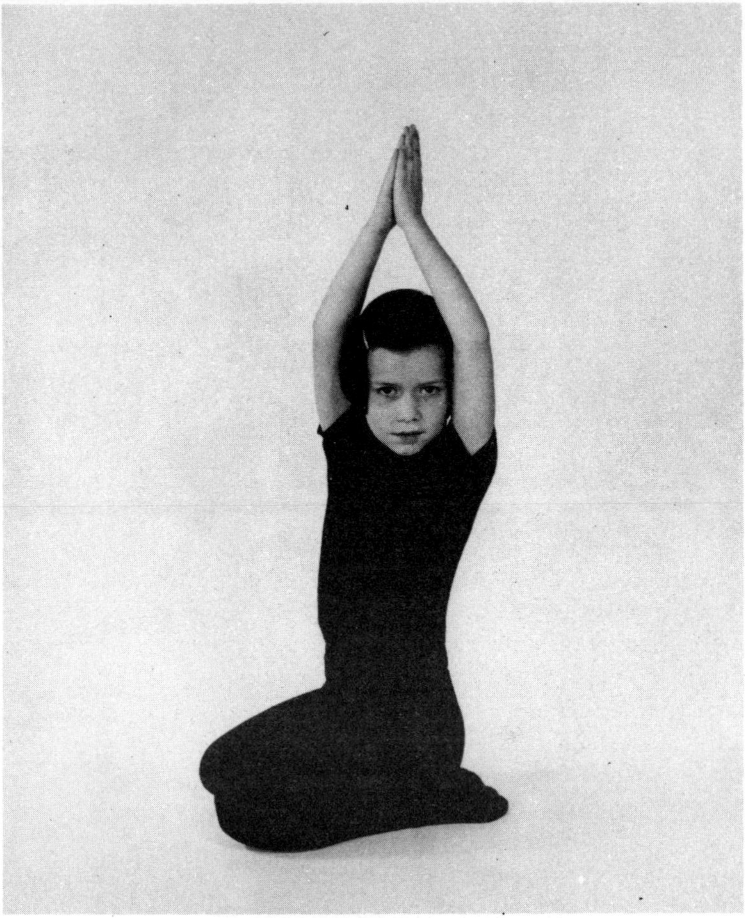

Sit on your heels and, breathing in, stretch both arms above your head with your palms together. Breathing out, twist your body, from the waist, to the right, breathing in, twist it back and breathing out, twist it to the left. Breathing in, twist it back and breathing out, lower your arms and rest your hands on your knee. After a breathing pause, repeat twice then rest on your back (savasana).

(Strengthens the back.)

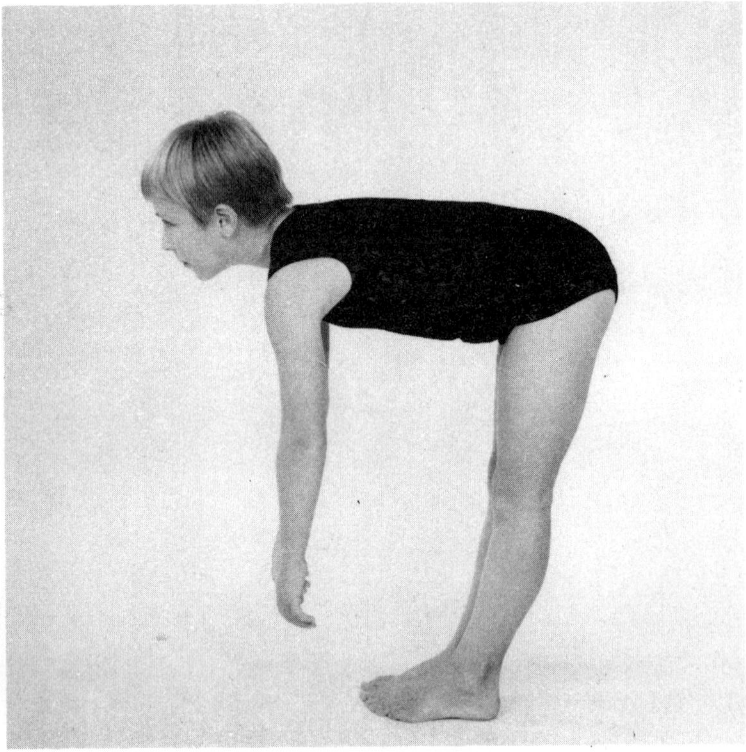

Stand upright, your feet together. Breathe in deeply. Breathing out bend forward so that your back and your legs are at right angles to one another. Your back should be straight and your arms hanging loosely at your sides. Breathing in, return to a normal standing position and breathe regularly. Repeat twice, then rest on your back (savasana).

(Strengthens the abdominal and back muscles.)

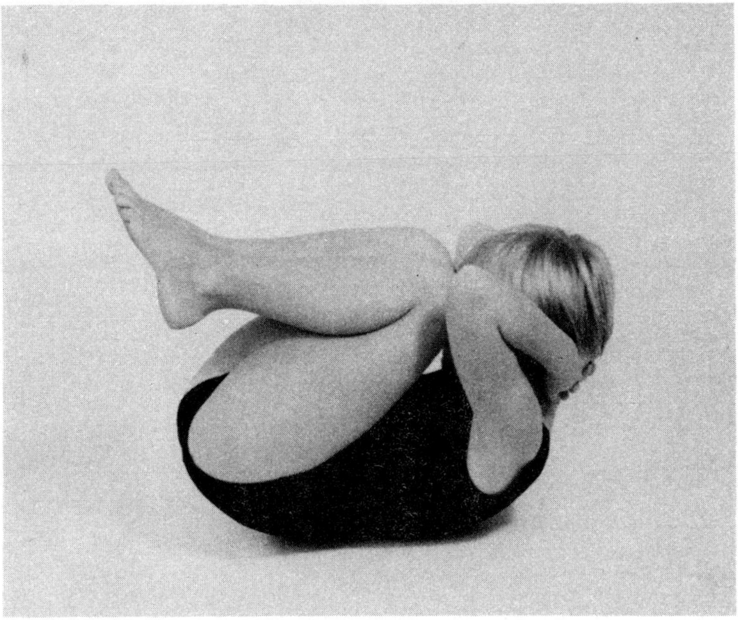

Lie on your back. Raise your arms so that your hands are supporting the back of your head. Breathe in deeply and peacefully. Breathing out, lift your head and pull up your knees so they are touching your forehead. Breathing in, lie back again and breathe peacefully. After a pause, repeat. Do the exercise three times in all and then rest on your back (savasana).

(Improves circulation).

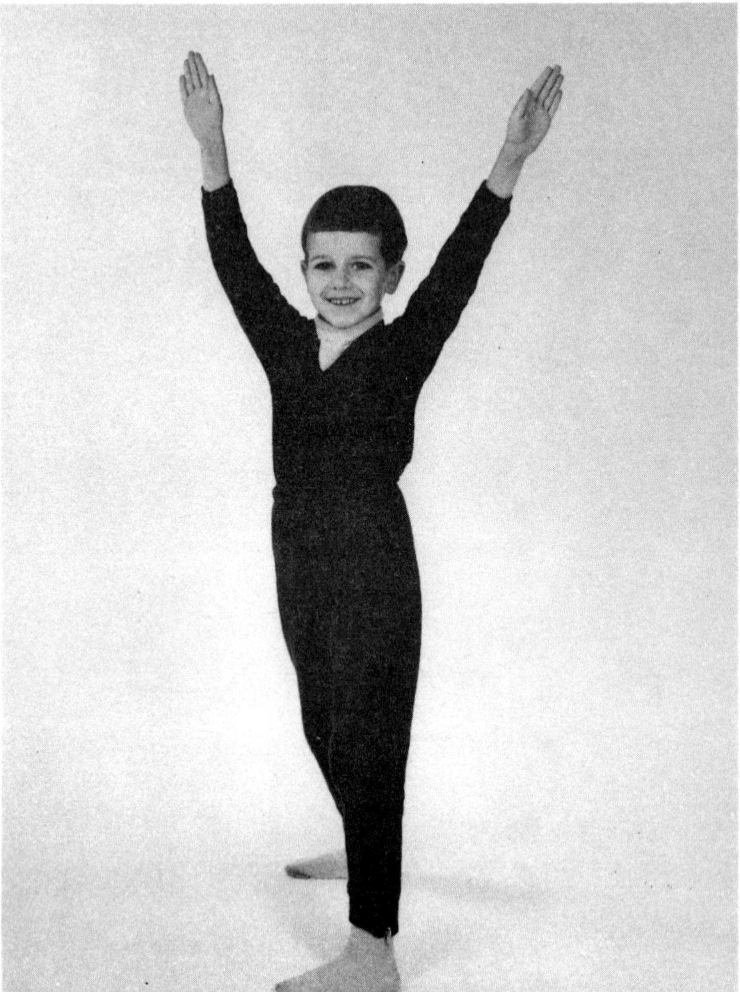

Stand with your legs apart. Breathing in, stretch both arms above your head. Breathing out, twist your body to the left and breathing in, twist it back. Breathing out, twist to the right, breathing in, back again. Breathe out and lower your arms. After a breathing pause repeat. Do this exercise three times in all.

(Strengthens the back.)

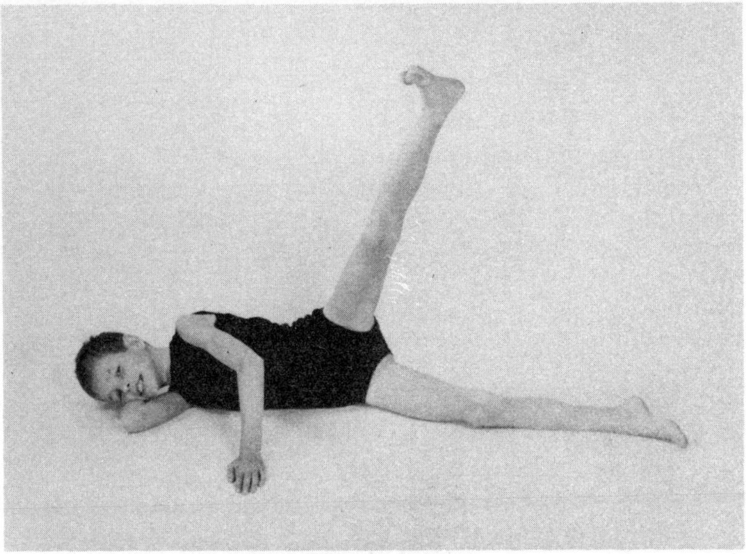

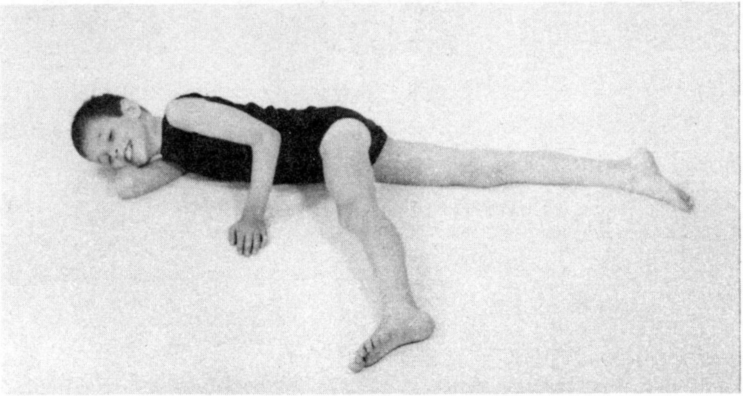

Lie on your right side, your right arm bent under your head, your left hand stretched out in front of your body. Breathing in, lift and stretch out your left leg, lowering it as you breathe out. Repeat twice. Then, breathing in, lift and stretch your left leg but this time as you breathe out, lower it so that it is almost at right angles to your body. Breathing in, raise it again and breathing out, return to your starting position. Repeat twice. Then repeat the entire exercise lying on your left side and moving your right leg. Afterwards rest on your back (savasana).

(Strengthens the abdominal and leg muscles.)

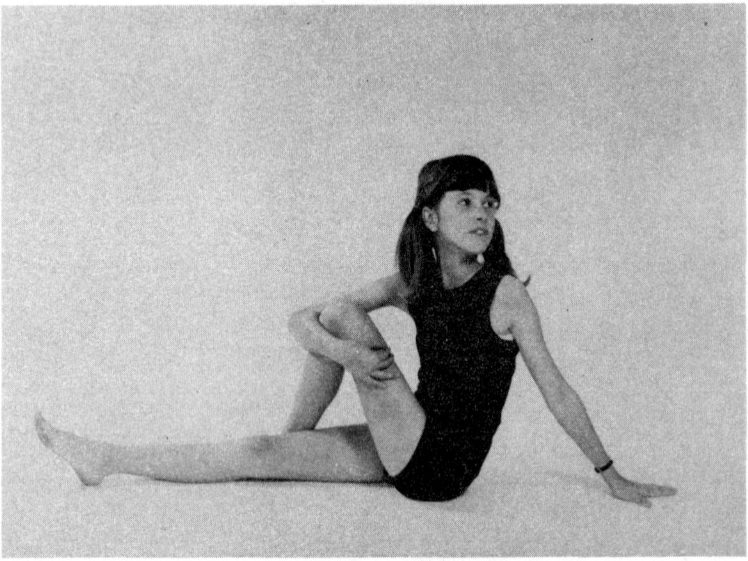

VAKRASANA

Sit with your legs stretched out in front of you. Cross your left leg over your right so your left foot is placed flat on the floor close to your right knee. Curl your right elbow round your left knee and draw your left shoulder back, supporting it with your left arm which is stretched out behind your body, the palm of your hand flat on the floor. Turn your head so you are looking over your left shoulder. Hold the pose while you calmly breathe in and out 3–5 times. Then reverse the position, repeating the exercise on your other side. Afterwards rest on your back (savasana).

(Promotes elasticity; strengthens the nerves.)

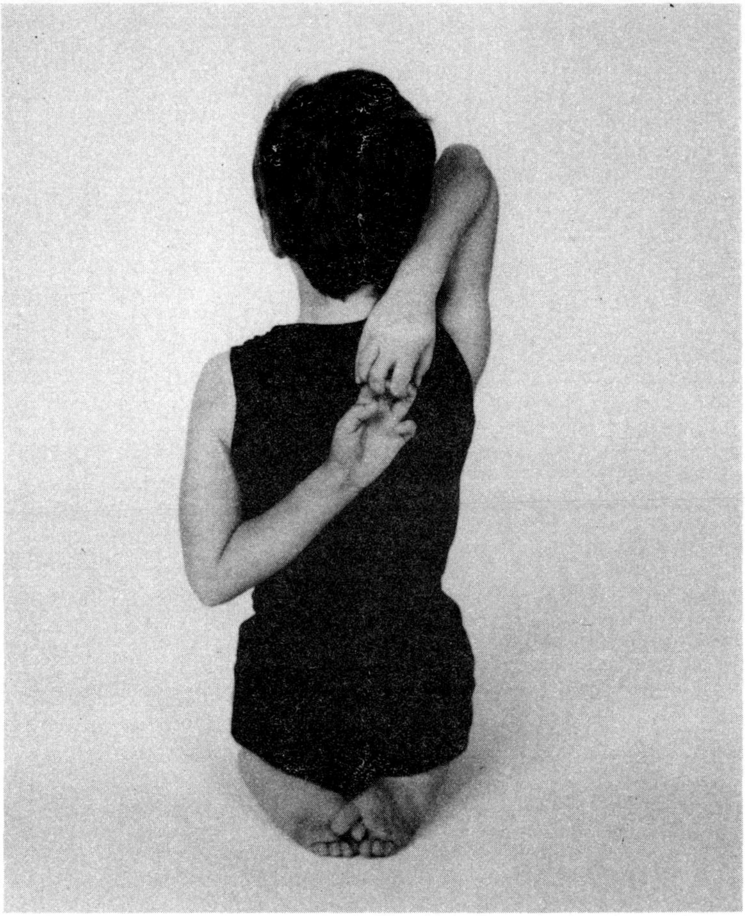

GOMUKHASANA

Sit on your heels. Bend your right arm down over your right shoulder and bring your left arm up to meet it, bend from about waist-level, so your hands join in the centre of your back. Hold the position long enough to breathe in and out slowly and then reverse it by bending your left arm down over your left shoulder and your right arm up from your waist.

(Strengthens the shoulder, arm, and back muscles.)

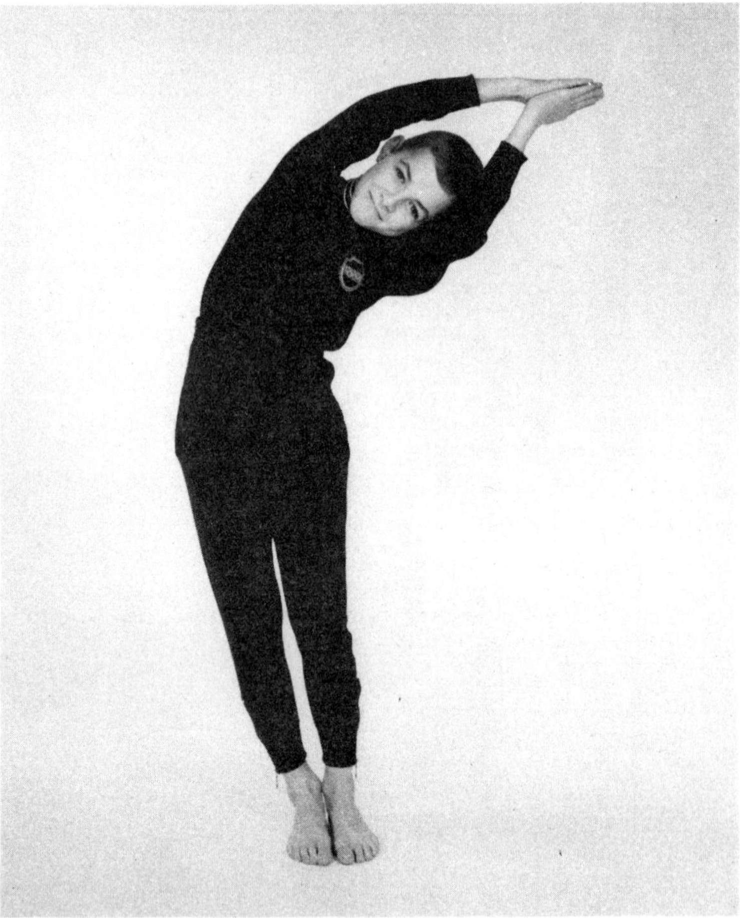

ARDHA CHANDRASANA I

Stand up straight with your feet together. Breathing in, raise your arms above your head and bring your palms together. Breathing out, bend over to the right. Breathe in and stand upright again and breathing out, bend over to the left. Breathe in and stand straight, and breathing out, lower your arms. After a pause repeat, doing the exercise three times in all on each side. Then rest on your back (savasana).

(Improves flexibility of the spine.)

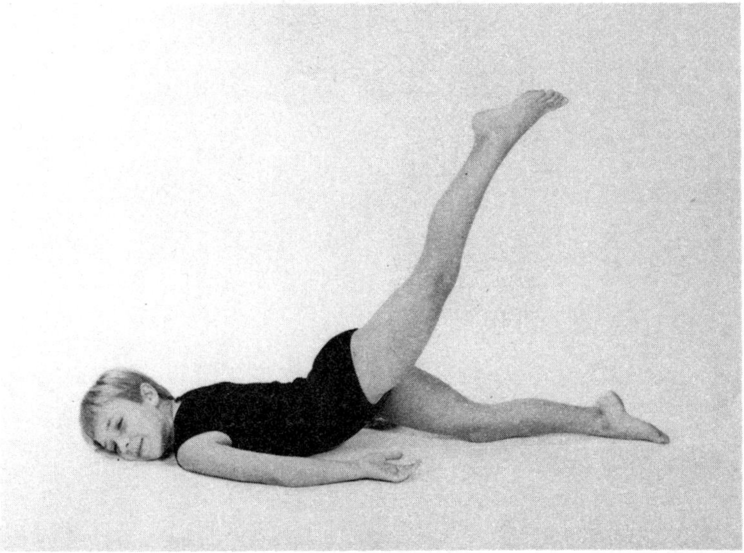

Lie on your back with your arms resting by your sides. Turn your head to the right and, breathing in, lift and stretch out your left leg. Breathing out, lower it again. Turn your head to the left and, breathing in, lift and stretch out your right leg. Breathing out, lower it, place your hands under your forehead and rest. Repeat twice.

(Good for the kidneys.)

Begin in the 'all-fours' position with your hands and knees on the floor. Breathing in, lift your right leg and stretch it out behind you; at the same time lift your head. Breathing out, lower your head and draw your right knee forward until it touches your forehead. Breathing in, lift your head and stretch your right leg out behind you. Then breathing out, return to the 'four-footed' stand. Repeat the whole exercise with your left leg. After a breathing pause repeat once more on both sides then rest sitting on your heels, bent forward so that your forehead is supported by your fists, placed one on top of the other.

(Strengthens the abdominal and leg muscles.)

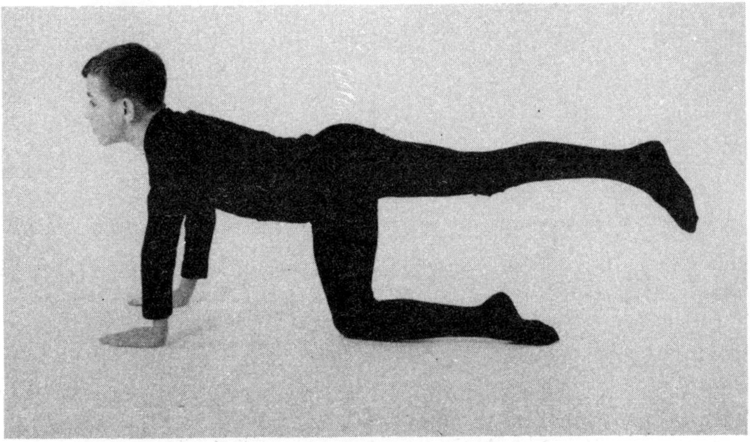

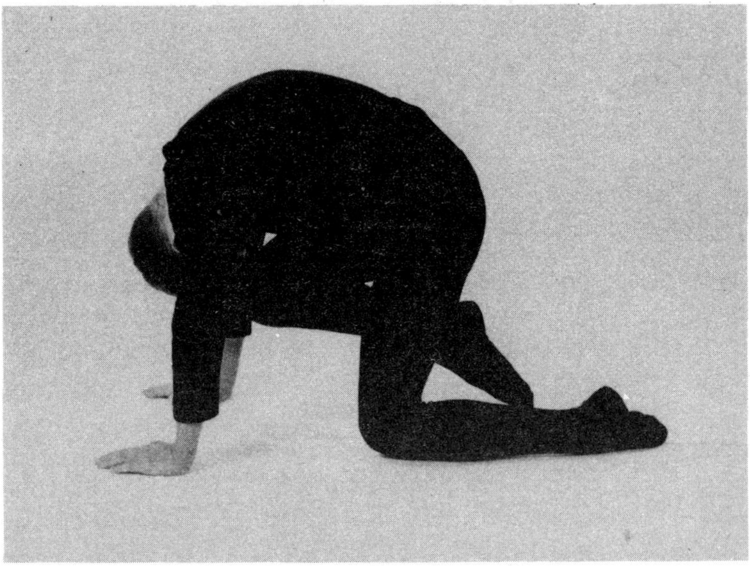

TRIKONASANA

Stand with your feet apart. Breathing in, lift your arms to shoulder height with your palms facing upwards. Breathing out, bend over until your left hand is touching your left foot, raise your right arm and turn your head so you are looking at your right hand. Breathing in, stand up straight, then repeat, bending to the right. After a breathing pause, repeat the entire exercise and then rest on your back (savasana).

(Strengthens the back muscles; invigorates the muscles on either side of the spine; encourages the elimination of toxins following infectious diseases.)

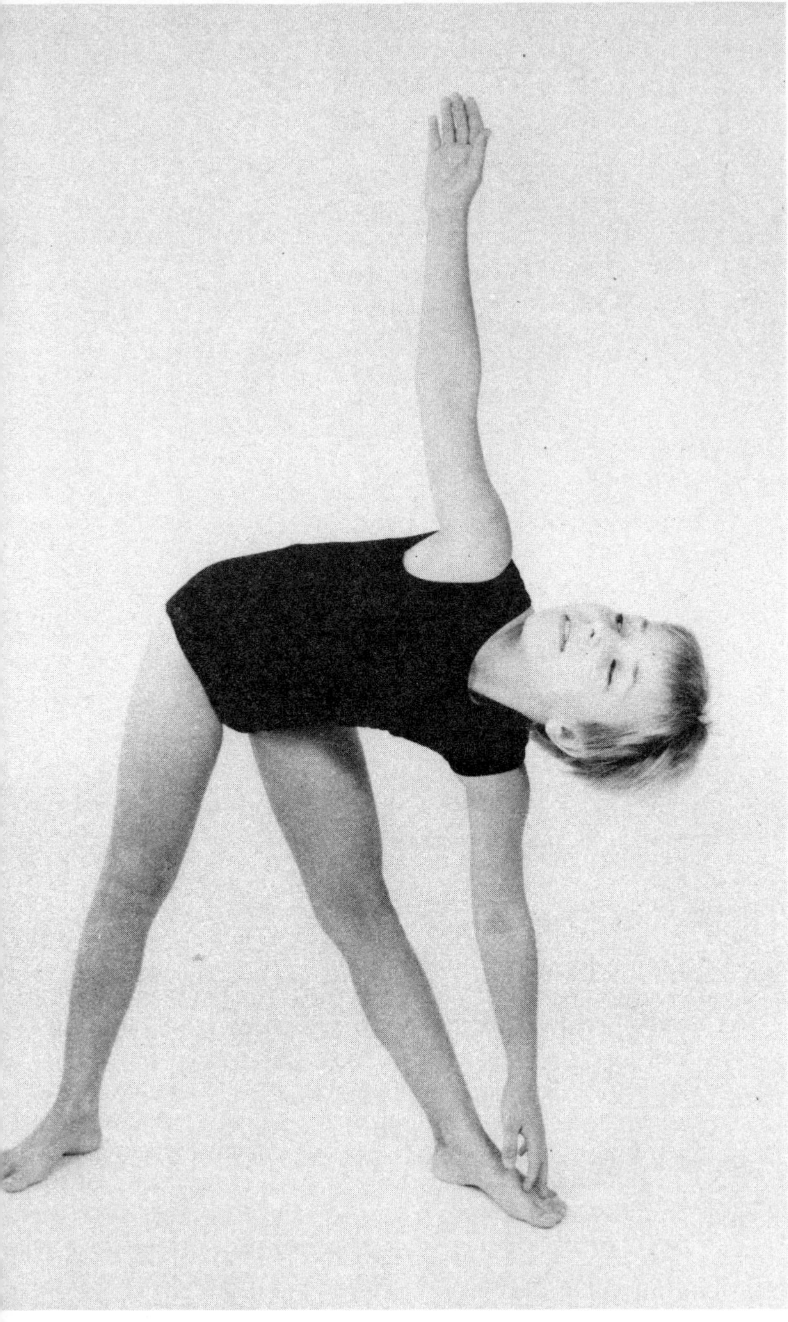

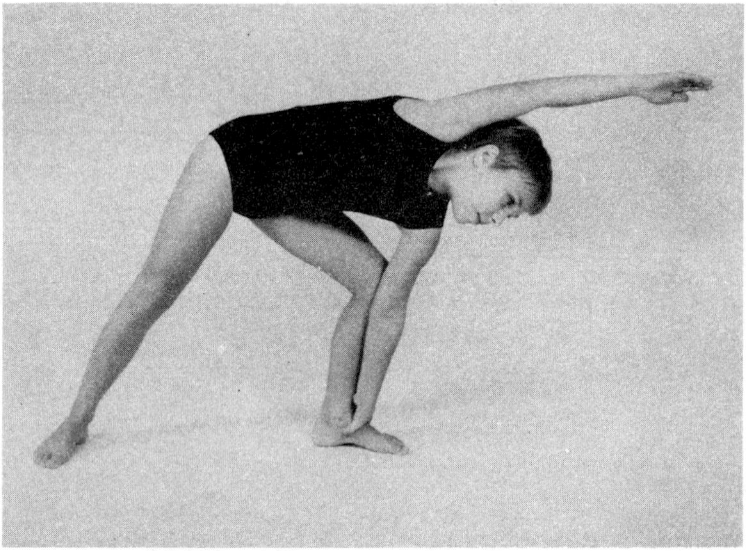

TRIKONASANA variation

Stand with your feet apart. Breathing in, raise your arms to shoulder height with your palms facing upwards. Breathing out, bend your left knee and bend over to the left until your left hand is touching your left foot. Your right arm should be stretched over your head parallel to the floor. Breathing in, stand up straight. Then repeat bending to the right. After a breathing pause, repeat the entire exercise and afterwards rest on your back (savasana).

(Strengthens the back muscles; invigorates the muscles on either side of the spine; encourages the elimination of toxins following infectious diseases.)

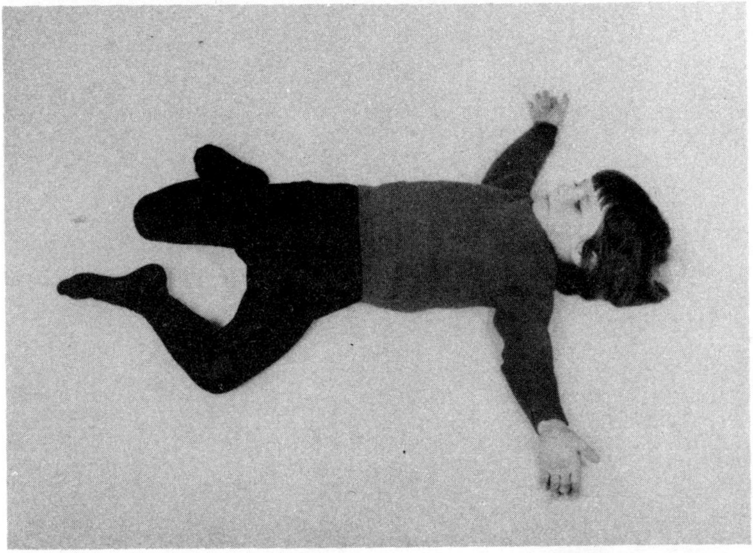

Twisting exercise

Lie on your back with your arms stretched out at shoulder level. Both legs should be bent and your feet wide apart on the floor. Without lifting your feet from the floor, tilt your knees over to the right until they are resting on the floor. Hold the position for about 30 seconds, breathing deeply and regularly. Raise your knees and then repeat the exercise by tilting them to the left. Return to the starting position, stretch out your legs and rest your arms by your sides. Repeat twice after a brief pause. Finally rest on your back (savasana).

(Improves elasticity especially of the lumbar region.)

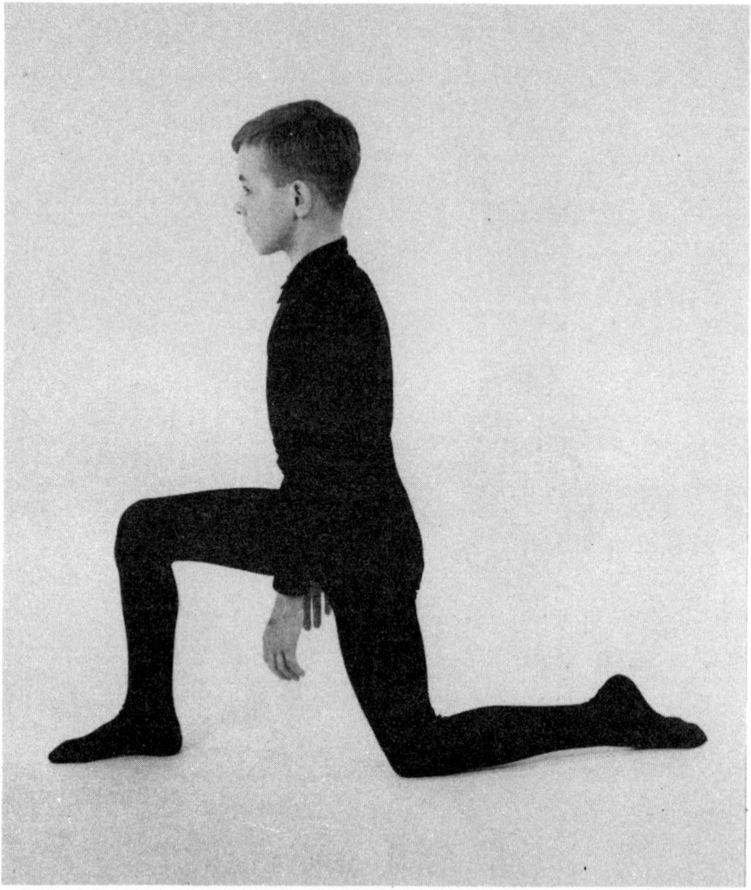

ARDHA-BHUDSHANGASANA

Kneel on your left knee with your right foot forward, your arms hanging loosely and relaxed. Breathe in deeply and relax ('full breathing'). Breathing out, transfer your weight from your left knee to your right foot, making sure that you keep your back straight. Breathing in, slowly return the weight to

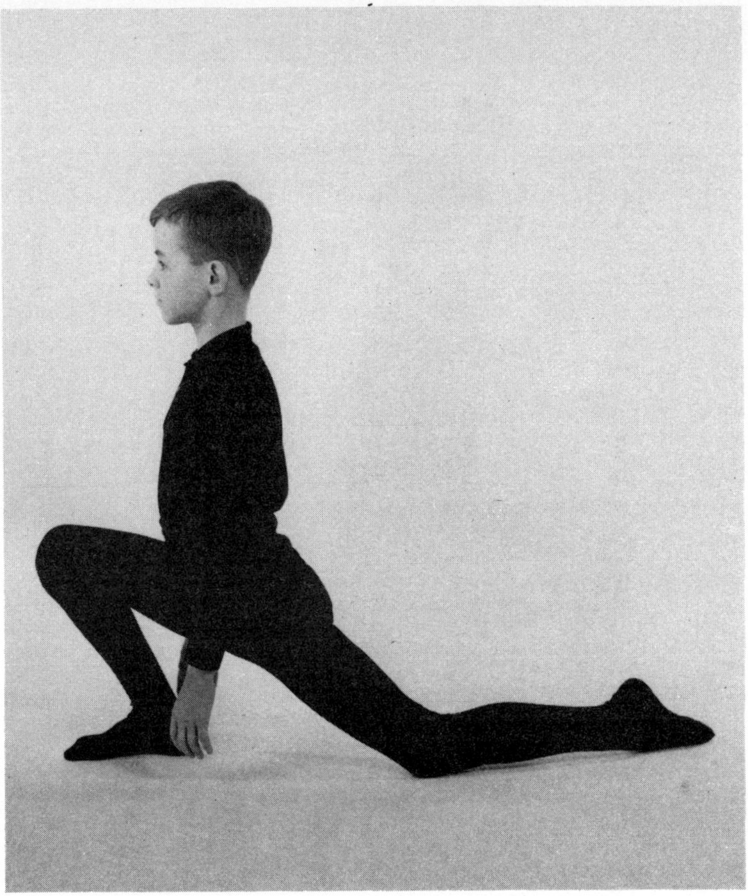

your left knee. Repeat twice. Then reverse the position of your feet and do the same thing transferring your weight from your right knee to your left foot and back again. Make sure that you also keep the heel of the foot that is in front, on the ground.

(Increases the suppleness and flexibility of the whole skeletal frame; prevents the formation of fatty deposits on the hips; improves sense of balance.)

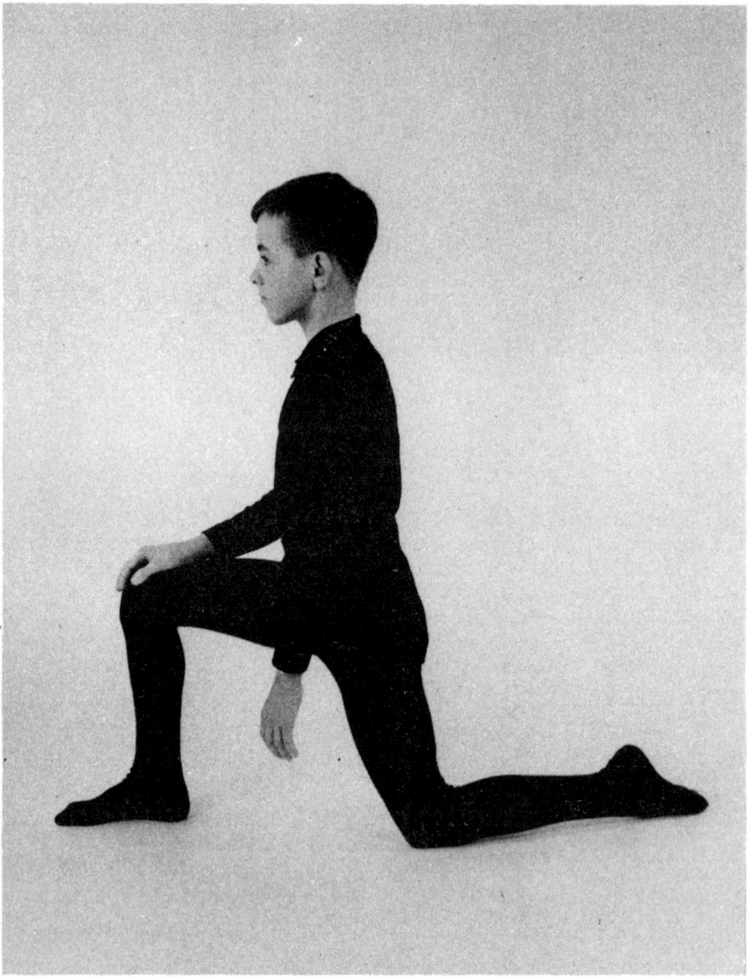

ARDHA-BHUDSHANGASANA

Kneel on your left knee, with your right foot forward and your right hand resting on your right knee. Breathe in deeply and relax ('full-breathing'). Breathing out, transfer your weight from your left knee to your right foot, simultaneously turning your body to the right (start turning at the small of your back, then your waist, shoulders and lastly your head). At the same time rest your left hand on your left leg. Breathing in, face forwards

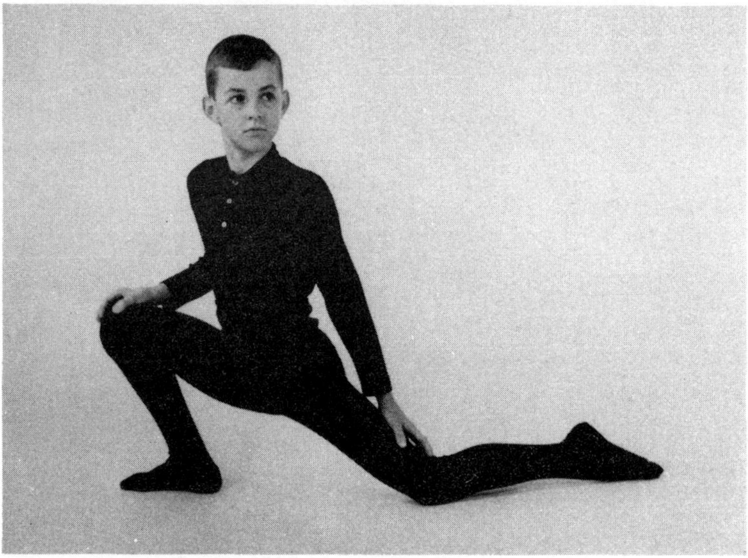

again, returning your weight to your left knee. Repeat twice. Then do the same exercise but in the reverse position: kneeling on the right knee with the left foot forward and twisting your body to the left. Make sure that you keep the heel of your leading foot firmly on the ground.

(Increases suppleness and elasticity of the skeleton; prevents the formation of fatty deposits on the hips; improves sense of balance.)

Section B exercises

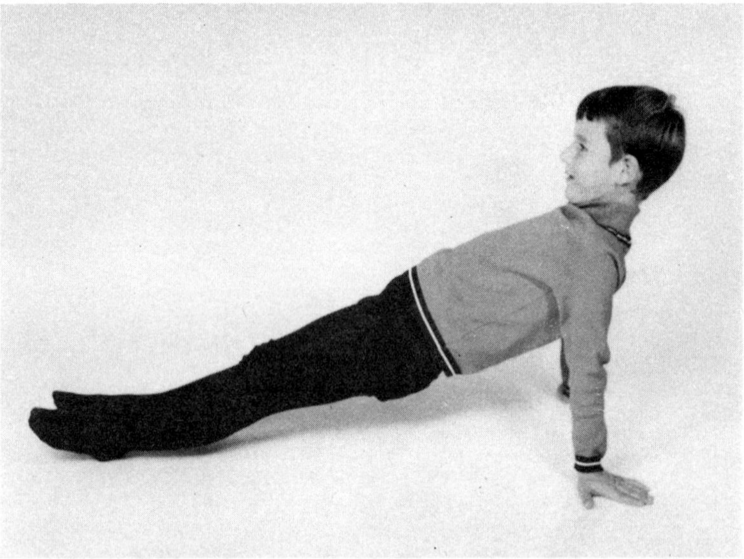

Sit with your legs stretched out in front of you. Breathing in, raise your body off the floor, supporting yourself on your hands (your arms should be straight and stretched out behind you). Breathing out, lower your body onto the floor. Repeat twice then rest on your back (savasana).

(Strengthens the spine and pelvis.)

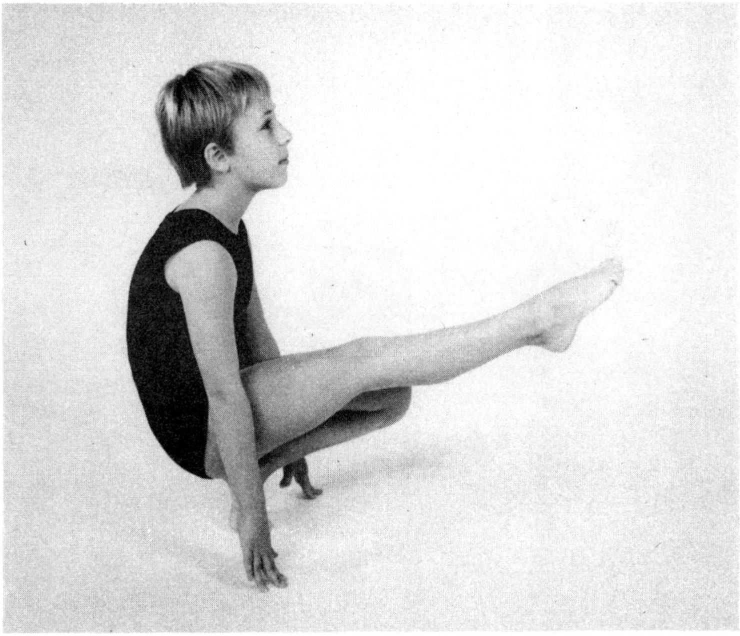

Sit in a squatting position, your hands on the floor and your fingers spread out. Stretch your right leg out in front of you so that it is completely straight and almost parallel to the floor. Your heels should not touch the floor. Return to your starting position and then repeat the same thing with your left leg. After a breathing pause repeat the whole exercise (i.e. stretching first your right and then your left leg) twice. Afterwards rest on your back (savasana).

(Strengthens the leg muscles.)

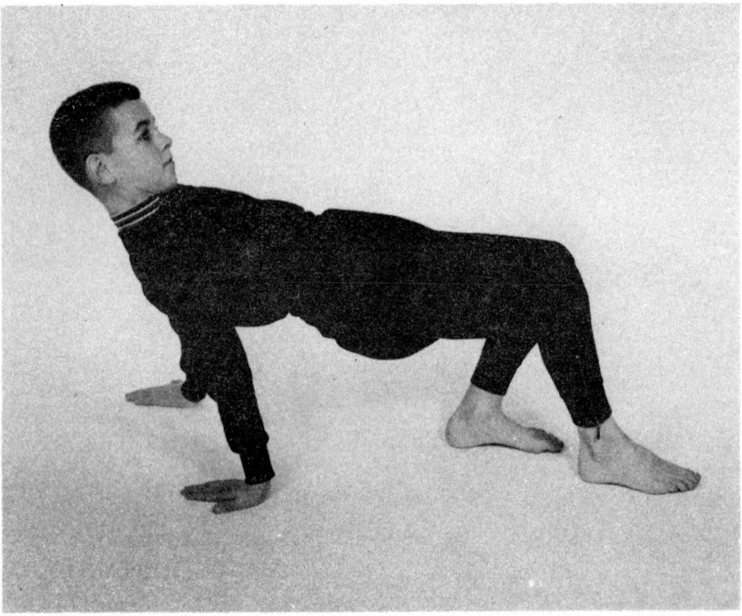

Sit with your knees together. Breathing in and supporting yourself on your hands, lift your pelvis and the small of your back off the floor. Then, breathing deeply and calmly, start to walk slowly on all fours (feet first). Take ten steps forwards and ten back. Then rest on your back (savasana).

(Strengthens the spine.)

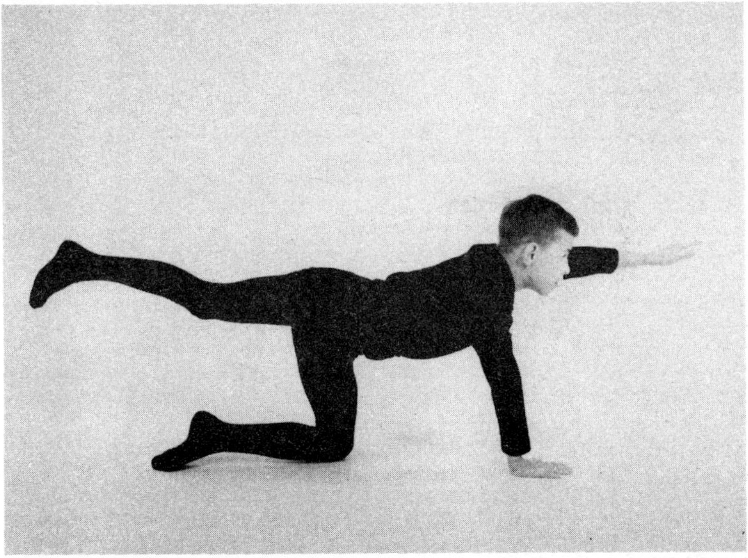

Adopt the ‘all-fours’ position (hands and knees on the floor). Breathing in, simultaneously raise your right leg and arm and hold them outstretched and parallel to the floor. Breathing out, return to your starting position. Breathing in, raise your left arm and leg in the same way. Breathing out, return to your original position. After a breathing pause repeat the whole exercise once more and then rest, sitting on your heels, bent forward, supporting your forehead with your fists.

(Improves balance.)

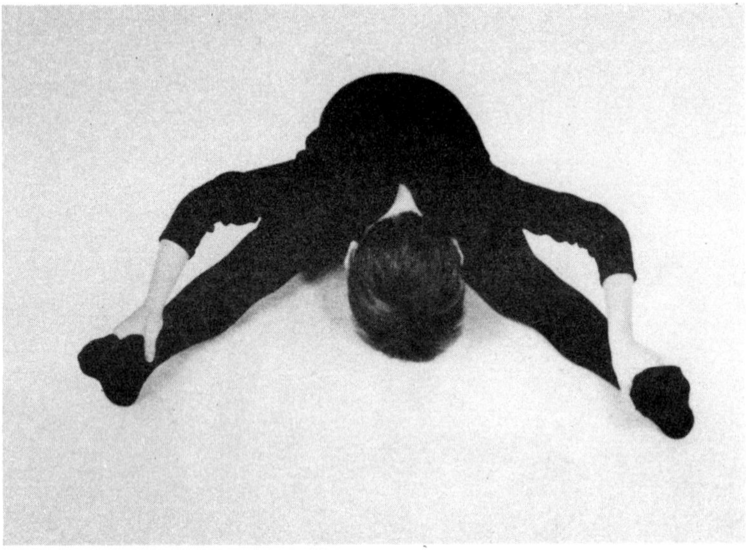

HASTHA-PADASANA

Sit with your legs wide apart. Breathe in deeply and then breathing out, bend forward. Hold on to your ankles and try to touch the floor with your forehead. After about five seconds, breathe in and sit up straight. Relax and breathe regularly. After a breathing pause, repeat twice. Then rest on your back (savasana).

(Strengthens the spine, small of the back, pelvis and legs.)

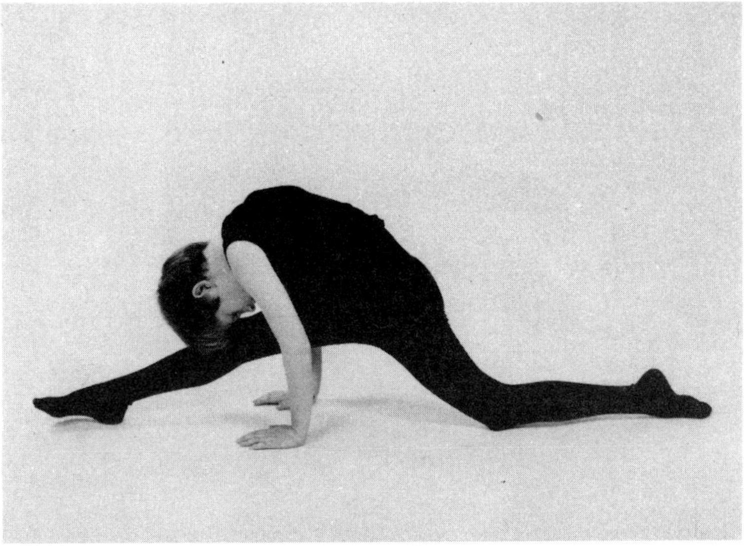

Adopt the 'all-fours' position (hand and knees on the floor). Breathe in calmly and deeply. Breathing out, push your right leg forward between your hands until your legs are wide apart, and rest your head on your right knee. Breathing in, lift your head and return to your starting position. After a breathing pause repeat the same thing with your left leg stretched forward. Then sit back on your heels, bent forward, supporting your head with your fists. Rest for a short time, then repeat the whole exercise twice. Afterwards rest on your back (savasana).

(Exercises all the joints; removes fatty deposits around the waist and midriff.)

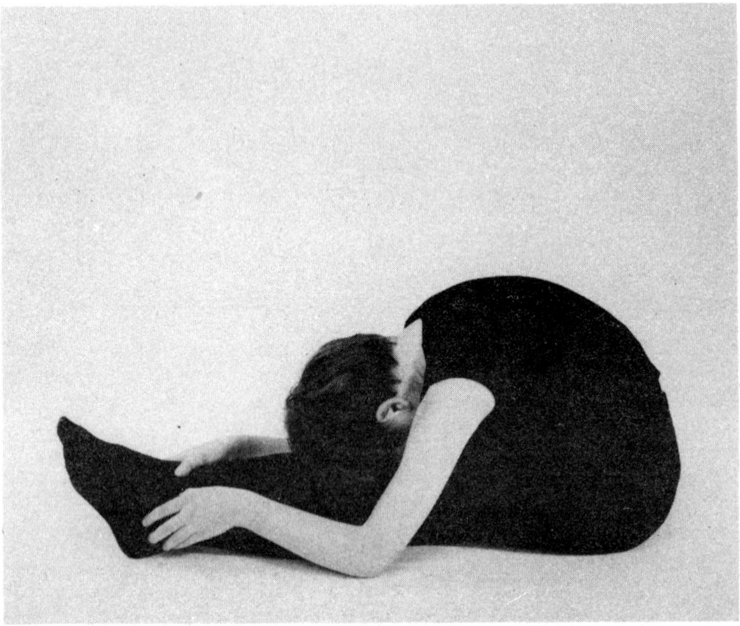

PASTSHIMOTANA

Lie on your back, your arms stretched out on the floor behind your head. Breathe in deeply and with your arms raised, slowly sit up. Breathing out, bend forward until your head is resting on your knees, and hold onto your ankles or toes. Your elbows should be touching the floor and your legs perfectly straight (don't bend your knees). Breathing in, sit up again and breathing out, slowly lie down on your back, your arms resting by your sides. After a breathing pause, repeat twice then rest on your back (savasana).

(Strengthens the back; benefits all abdominal organs; stabilizes health.)

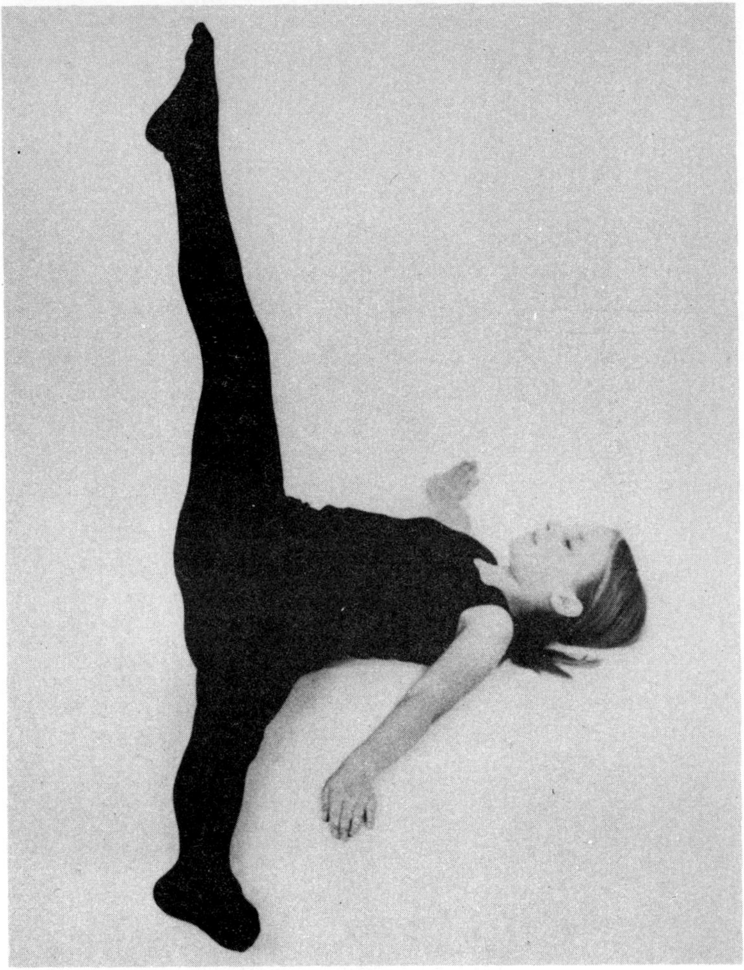

Lie on your back, your arms stretched out at shoulder level, your palms facing downwards. Breathing in, raise both legs so your toes are pointing to the ceiling. Breathing out, lay your left leg on the floor at a right angle to your body. Breathing in, raise it again. Repeat, raising and lowering your right leg. After a breathing pause lying on your back, repeat the entire exercise twice. Afterwards, rest in the savasana position.

(Strengthens abdominal and leg muscles.)

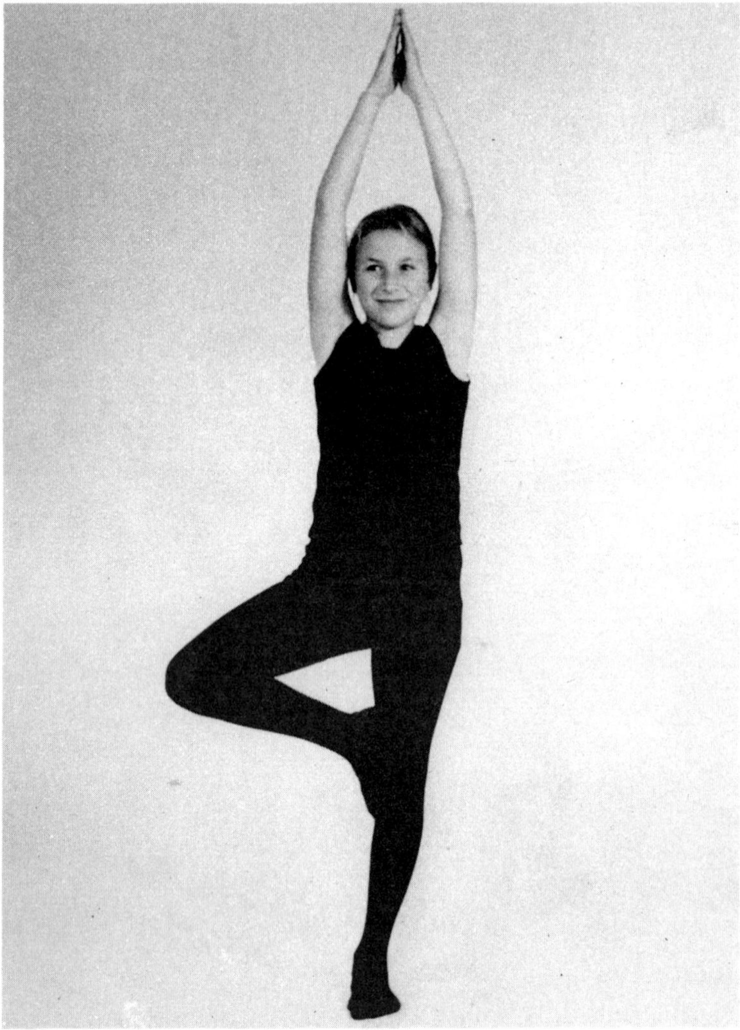

TREE POSITION

Stand on your right leg, your left foot against your right knee. Stretch your arms above your head, keeping your palms together, and breathe calmly and regularly. Hold the position for 30 seconds and then change legs. After a breathing pause, repeat twice, then rest on your back (savasana).

(Improves balance.)

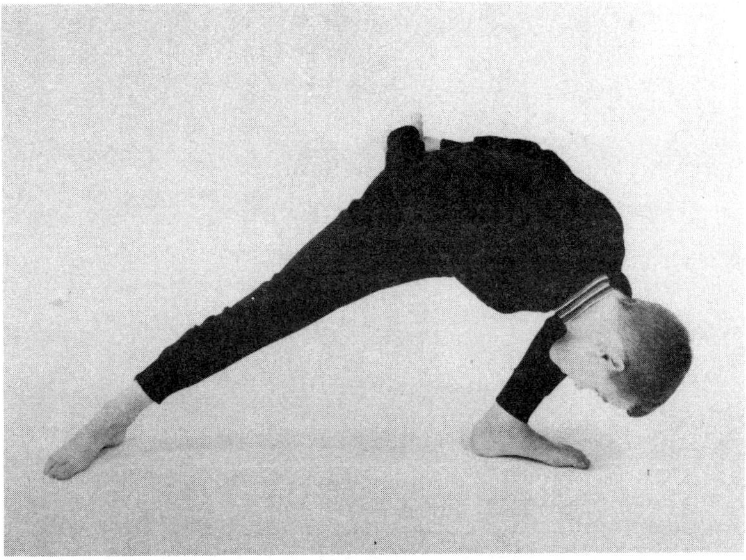

STRANGUSTHASANA

Stand with your feet wide apart. Breathing in, fold your hands behind your back. Breathing out, bend both your left knee and your body from the waist (as low as you can) so that your head is almost touching the floor. Breathing in, slowly stand up straight and then breathing out, bend to the right. Breathing in, straighten up again, and after a short breathing pause, repeat the entire exercise once more, bending first your left and then your right knee. Afterwards, relax on your back (savasana).

(Strengthens the pelvic and leg muscles; improves flexibility.)

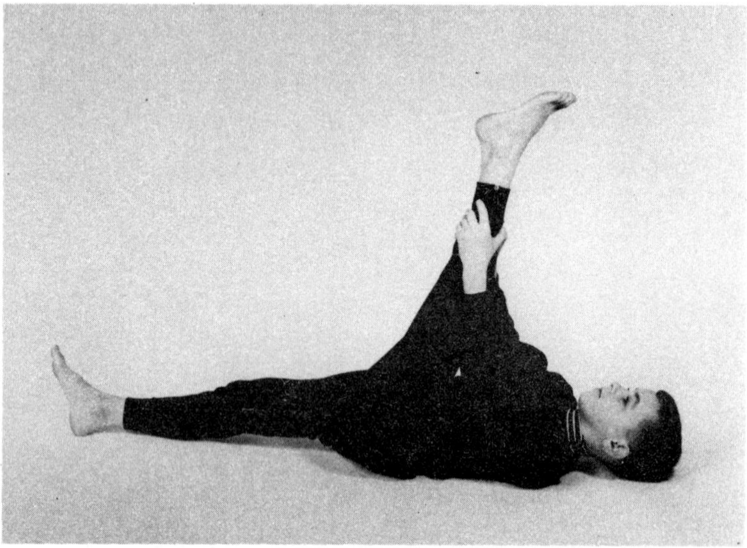

Lie on your back and breathe in deeply. Breathing out, raise and stretch your left leg. Hold on to it with both hands and try to draw it closer to your body. Breathing in, lower it to the floor. Breathing out, raise and stretch your right leg, and breathing in, rest lying on your back. Continue to breathe peacefully. After a pause, repeat the exercise twice and afterwards rest in the savasana position.

(Strengthens the abdominal and leg muscles.)

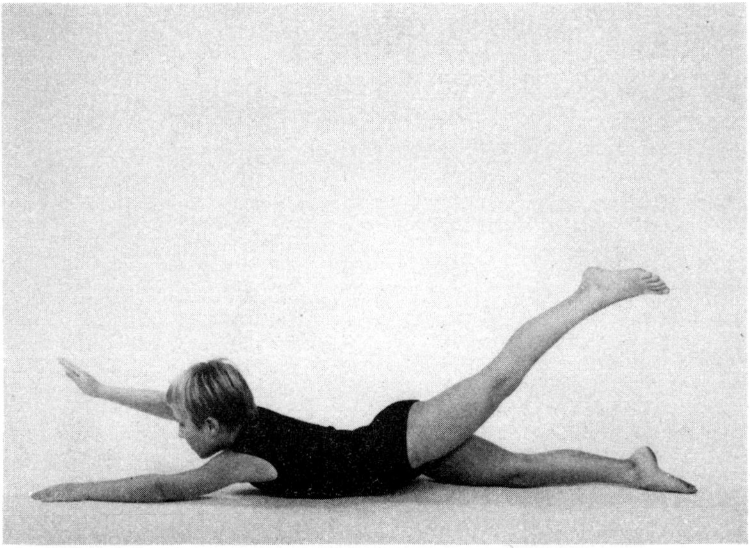

Lie on your front, your arms stretched out in front of you. Breathing in, raise your right arm and left leg from the floor. Breathing out, lower them, and breathing in again, raise your left arm and right leg. Breathing out, lower them, place your hands under your forehead and rest. Repeat twice.

(Increases elasticity; strengthens the back.)

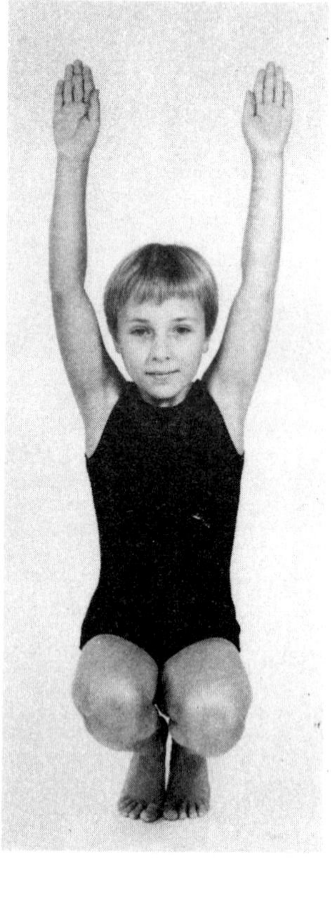

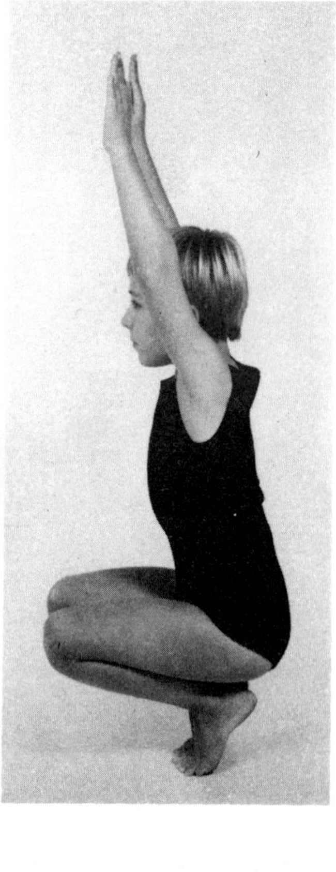

Stand up straight. Breathing in, raise your arms above your head and stand on your toes. Breathing out, bend your knees and squat on the floor. Breathing in, stand up straight (still on your toes) and breathing out, lower your heels to the floor and your arms to your sides. After a breathing pause, repeat once more. Then rest on your back (savasana).

(Strengthens the foot and leg muscles; improves balance.)

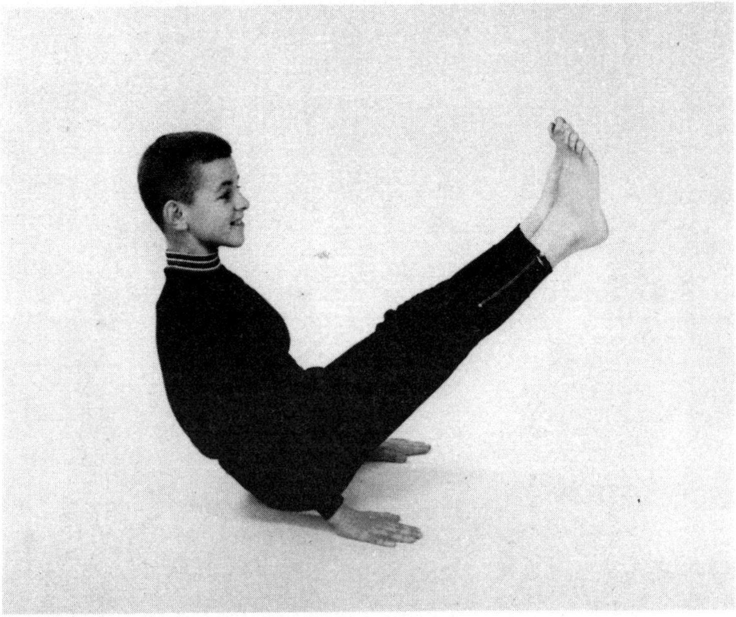

VADSHROLI-MUDRA

Sit with your knees together, your hands on the floor at your sides. Breathing in, raise your legs off the floor and hold the position breathing regularly for 20 seconds. Then lower your feet to the floor. Rest your forehead on your knees and wrap your arms round them. Relax and then repeat twice. Afterwards rest on your back (savasana).

(Develops stamina, determination and will-power).

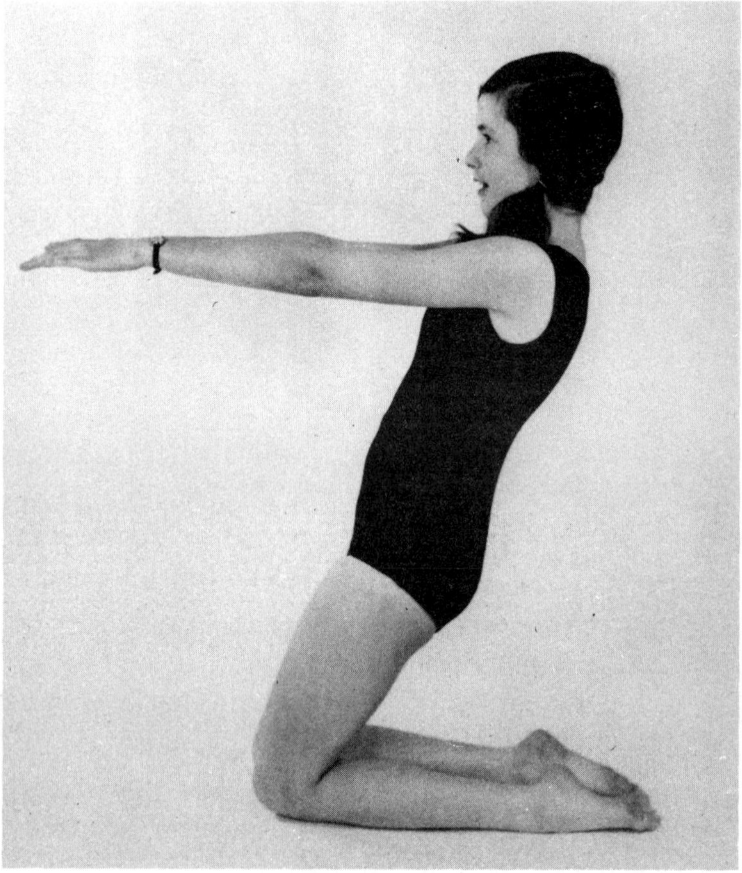

Kneel on the floor. Breathing in, raise both arms to shoulder height and breathing out, bend over backwards a little way. Breathing in, straighten up, and breathing out, lower your arms. Repeat twice, then rest on your back (savasana).

(Strengthens the thigh muscles and spine.)

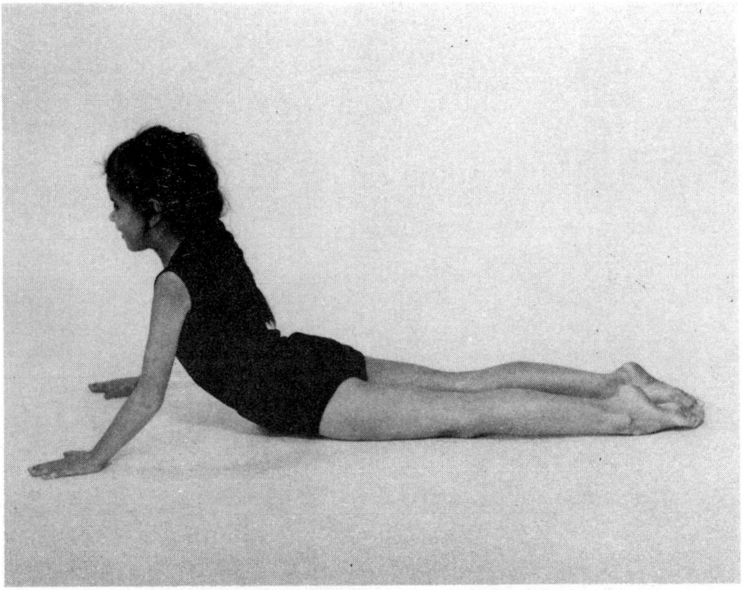

BHUDSHANGASANA

Lie on your front with your hands on the floor under your shoulders. Breathing in, slowly raise your head and then (your back muscles taking the strain) your shoulders and trunk. Be careful not to use your arms to push yourself up although you can let them take enough of the weight to prevent yourself slipping back. If it is not too great a strain, hold the position for 7–12 seconds without breathing. Then breathing out, slowly return to your starting position and rest with your hands under your forehead. After a breathing pause, repeat twice. Then rest on your back (savasana).

(Good for the kidneys; strengthens the spine and nervous system.)

NB: Not for anyone with an over-active thyroid gland.

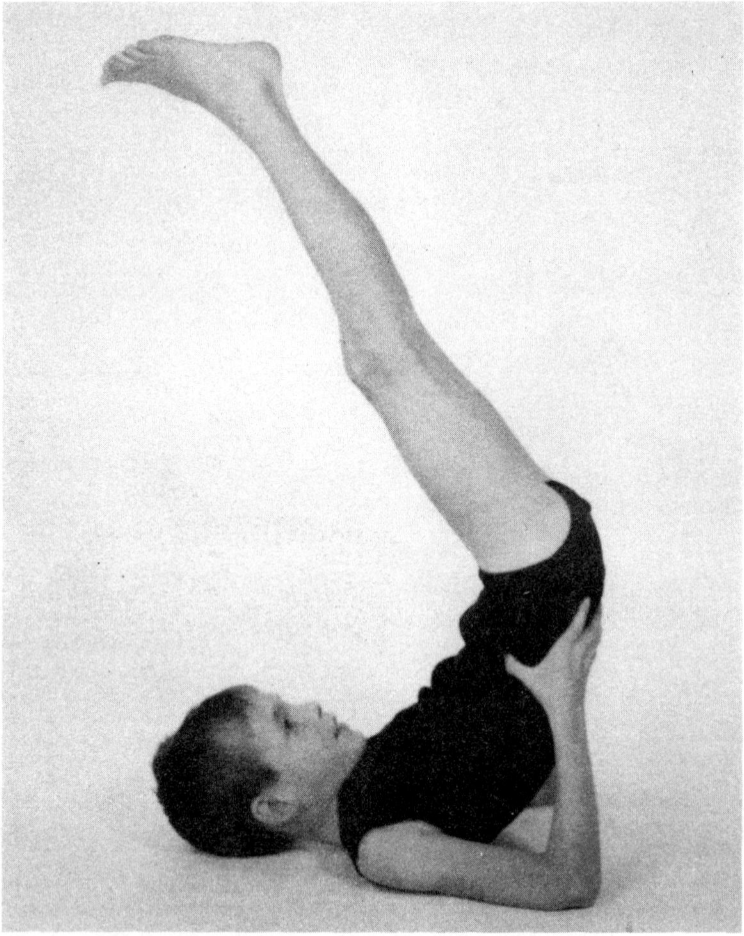

VIPARITAKARANI

Lie on your back. Breathing in, raise your legs and pelvis off the floor, supporting yourself with your hands under your hips. Hold the position (while diaphragm-breathing) as long as is comfortable. Then slowly bring your legs down to the floor and rest in the savasana position. Make sure that when you lower your legs, your head and shoulders remain on the floor.

(Strengthens the thyroid gland).

NB: This exercise is not recommended for anyone with damaged neck vertebrae.

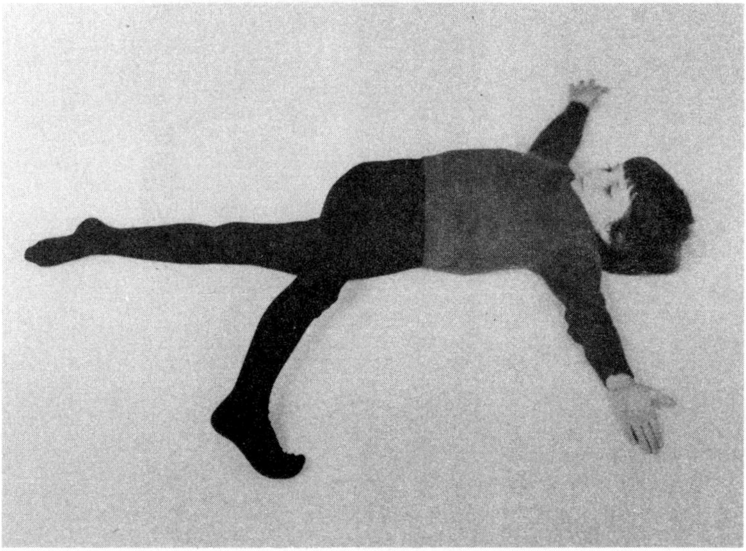

Twisting exercise

Lie on your back, your arms outstretched at shoulder level. Breathing in, lift up your right leg and breathing out, bring it down to the floor on your left side. Breathing in, lift it again, and breathing out, return to your starting position. Do the same thing with your left leg. Repeat twice then rest on your back (savasana).

(Increases flexibility; strengthens the abdominal and leg muscles.)

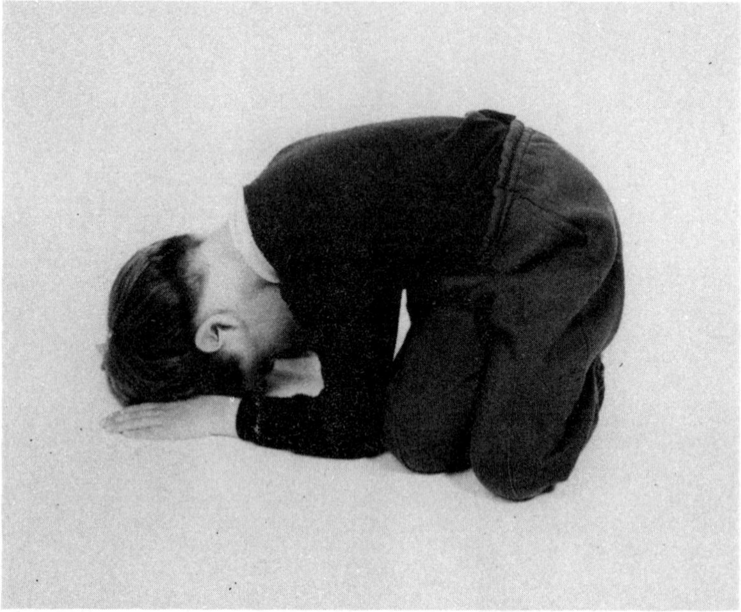

Twisting exercise

Sit on your heels, your hands on your thighs. Breathe in deeply and calmly. Breathing out, twist your body from the waist to the right and bend forward so that your hands, elbows and forhead are resting on the floor. Breathing in, sit up and twist your body back so you are facing straight ahead. Breathing out, twist to the left. After a breathing pause, repeat. Then rest on your back (savasana).

(Strengthens the back; increases elasticity.)

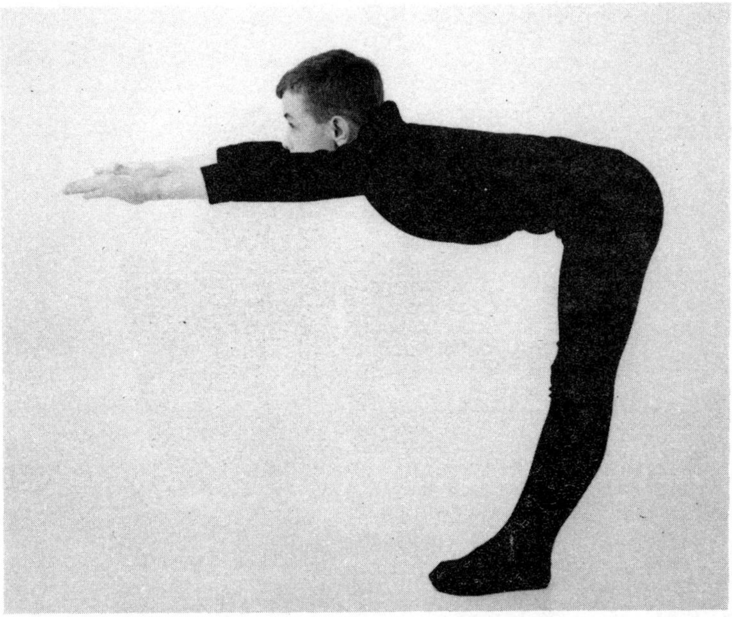

Stand with your feet together. Breathing in, stretch your arms above your head and breathing out, bend forward so that your arms and your body from the waist upwards are parallel to the floor. As you bend over push your bottom out behind you. Breathing in, stand straight and breathing out, lower your arms. Repeat twice. Then rest on your back (savasana).

(Strengthens the spinal column and small of the back.)

Section C exercises

PADMASANA (*Lotus position*)

Preliminary exercise: sit on the floor, your legs stretched out in front of you. Bending your right knee, place your right foot on your left thigh. Hold the position for as long as is comfortable. Stretch your right leg out again and bend your left knee, placing your left foot on your right thigh. Be patient and don't try to force your legs into position. When you can do this easily without any discomfort in your ligaments and tendons, you can try the lotus position:

Sit on the floor and lay your right foot on your left thigh close to your body. Then crossing your left leg over your right, place your left foot on your right thigh. Rest your hands on your knees, close your eyes and breathe slowly and deeply. Hold the position for as long as is comfortable.

(Calms the nervous system; stabilizes health.)

Make sure that when you are sitting in this position, your back, neck and head form a straight line.

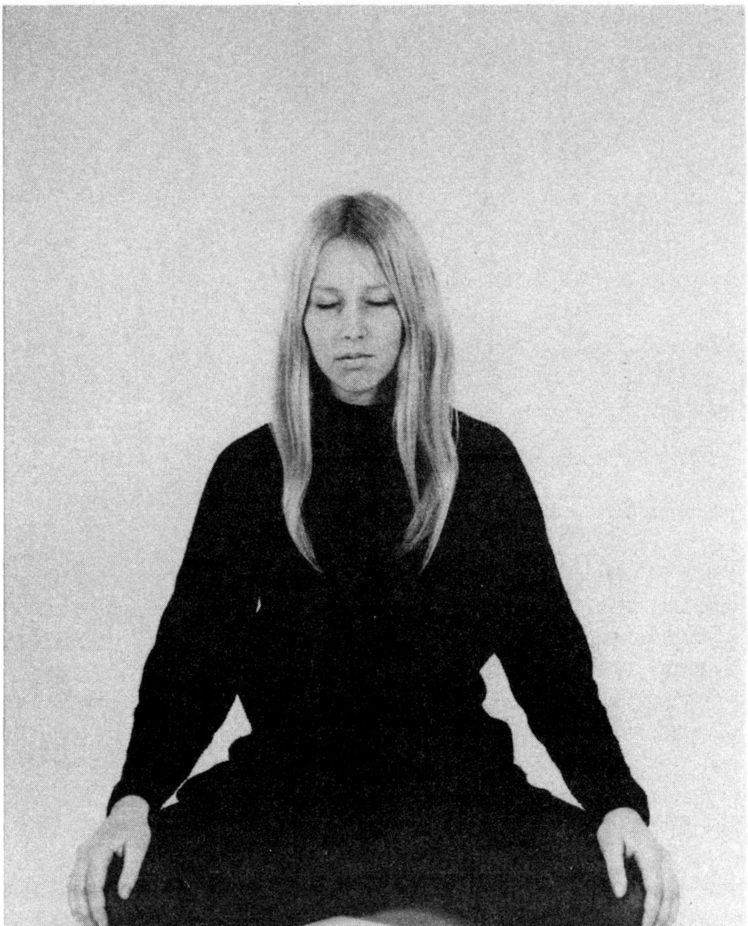

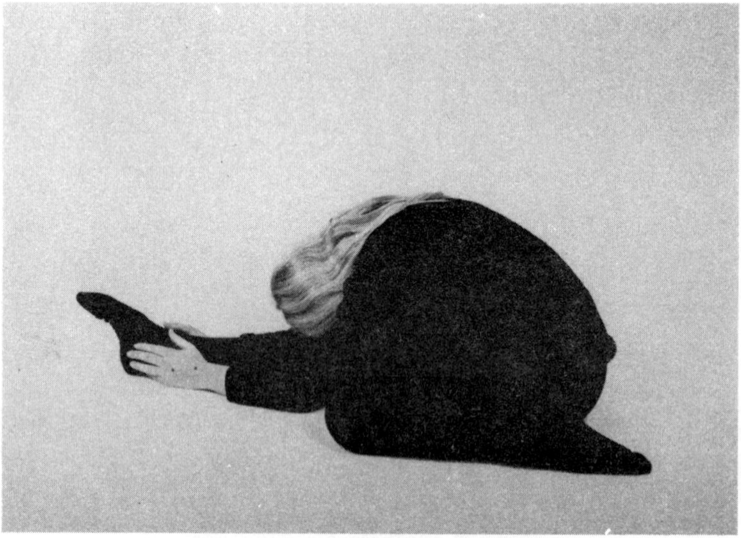

Sit with your legs stretched out in front of you. Then bend your left leg into the position shown in the picture. Breathing out, bend over your right knee and with your elbows on the floor, hold your right ankle. Breathing in, sit up again and after a breathing pause, repeat. Do the same thing with your left leg stretched and your right leg bent. Afterwards rest on your back (savasana).

(Increases flexibility; improves health.)

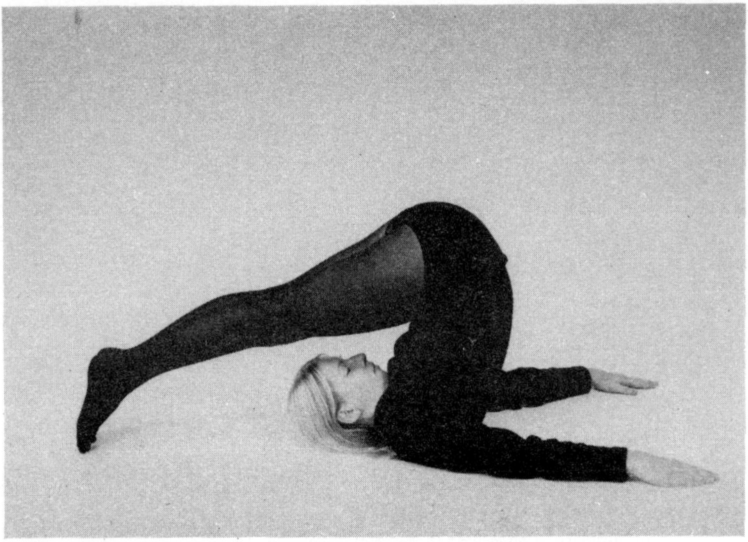

HALASANA

Lie on your back with your arms by your sides and your palms facing downwards. Slowly breathing in, raise your legs to the 'Roman Candle' position (VIPARITAKARANI). Then breathing out, lower your feet over your head to the floor. Breathing slowly, hold the position for as long as is comfortable. Then lift your legs back over your head and rest on your back (savasana).

(Promotes the development of the spine.)

NB: This exercise is not recommended for anyone with damaged neck vertebrae.

USTRASANA

Sit on your heels and hold your ankles. Breathing in, raise your pelvis and the small of your back quite high off the ground and hold the position, breathing deeply for 5–10 seconds. Then sit on your heels, bend forward and support your head on your fists placed one on top of the other. After relaxing in this position, repeat twice and then rest on your back (savasana).

(Removes fatty deposits on the hips and abdomen).

NB: Not for anyone with an over-active thyroid gland.

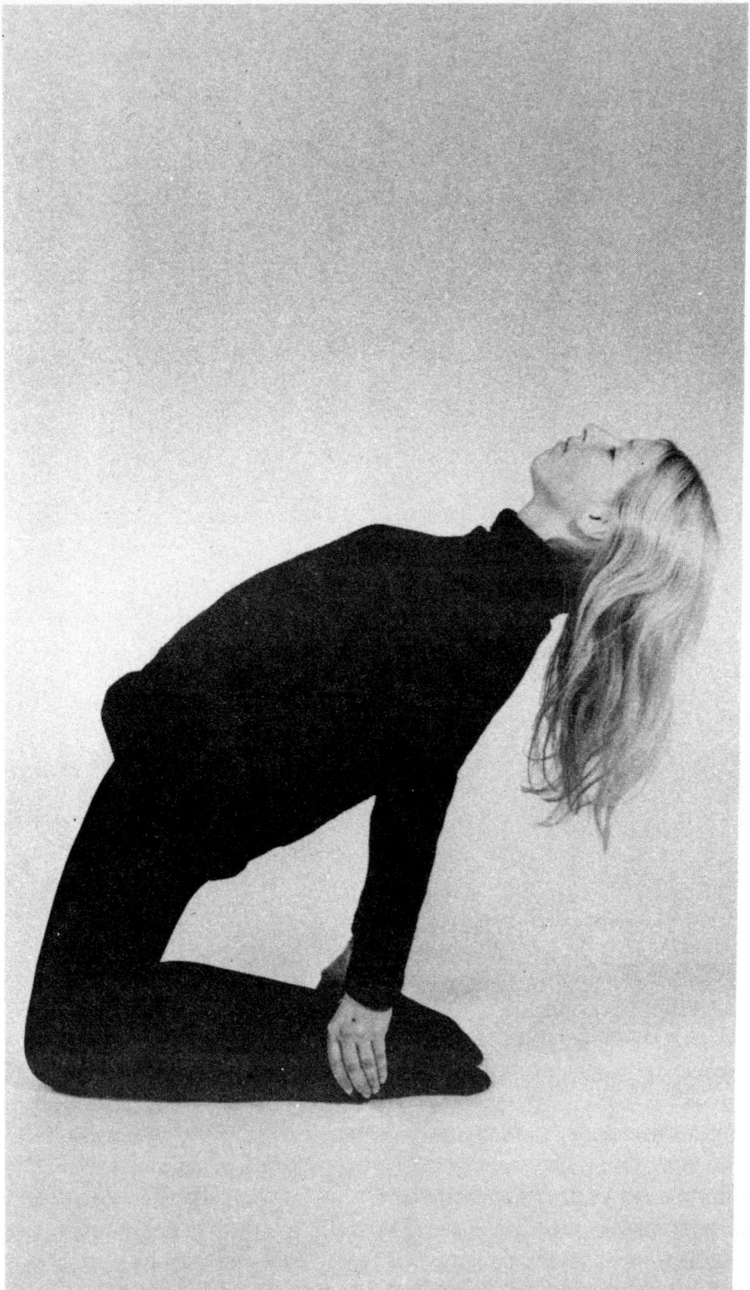

KAA-KAASANA

Squat on your toes, your legs apart. Put your hands on the floor in front of your feet and supporting your knees on your elbows, let your upper arms and elbows take your weight. Then slowly try to raise your feet from the ground. After a breathing pause, repeat twice then rest on your back (savasana).

(Improves sense of balance.)

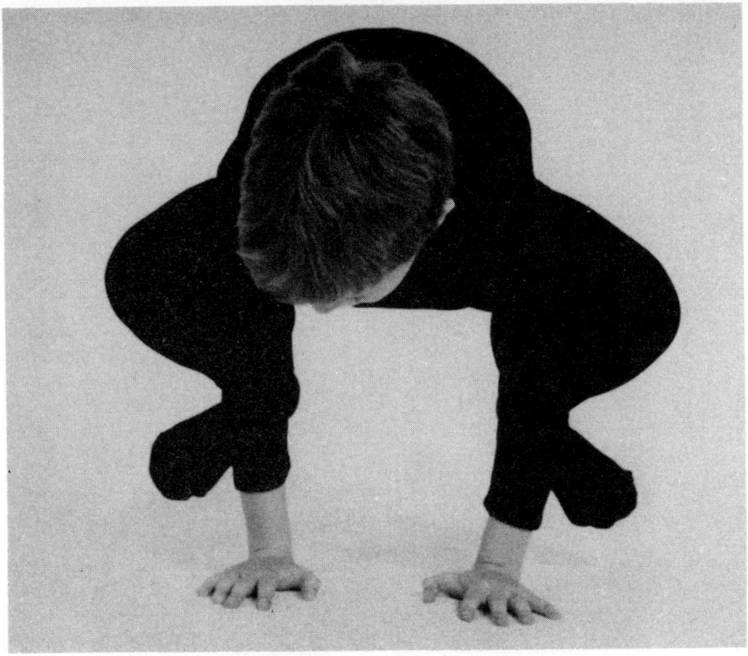

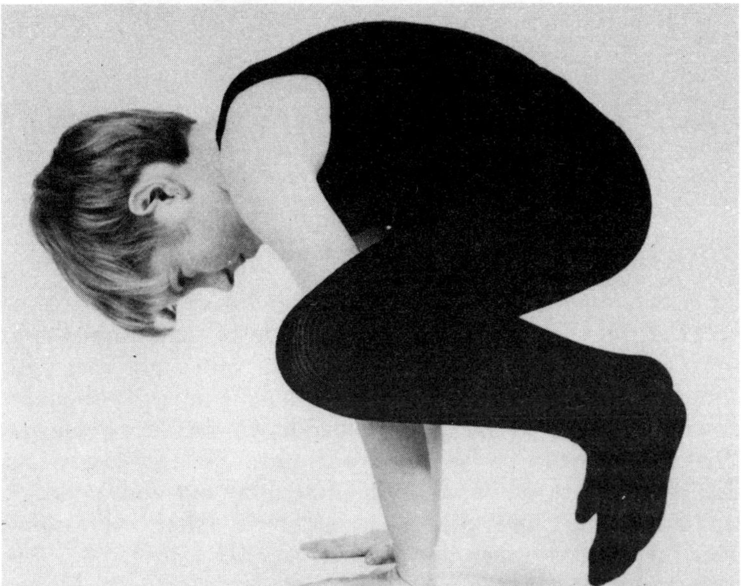

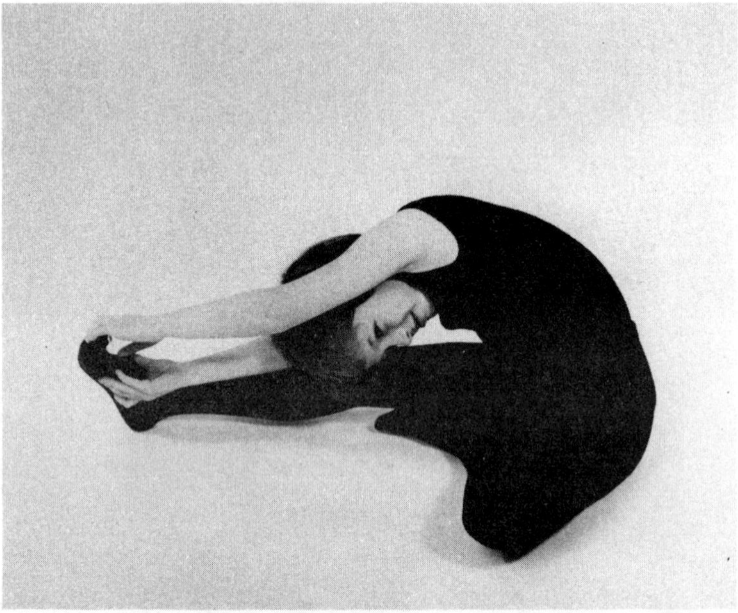

DSHANUSIRASANA (horizontal)

Sit with your legs apart. Bend your left leg so that the sole of your left foot is resting against the inside of your right thigh. Bend forward over your right leg. Clasp your right foot with both hands and at the same time, turning your right shoulder down towards your right leg, let your left shoulder come up. Your head should be between your arms. Breathe slowly and deeply. Sit up slowly and do the same thing but with your left leg outstretched and your right leg bent. After a breathing pause, repeat twice then rest on your back (savasana).

(Increases will-power.)

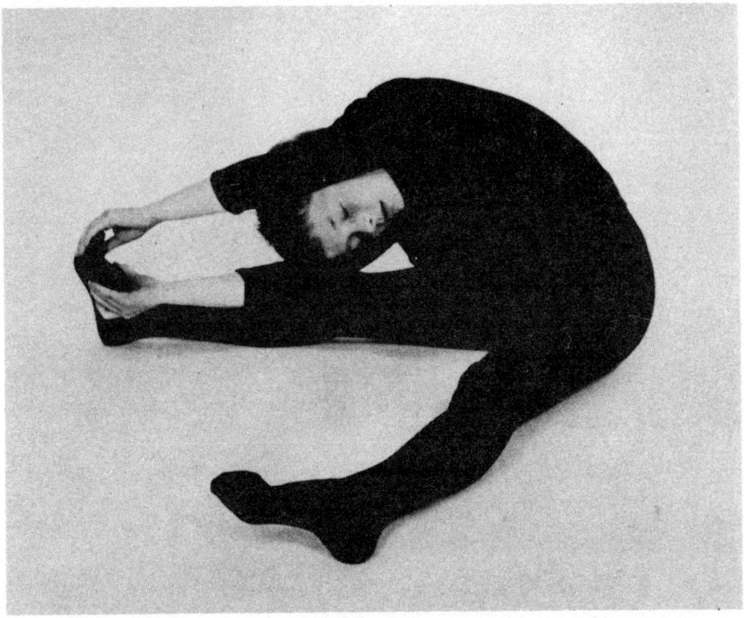

DSHANUSIRASANA (variation)

Sit with your legs apart. Bend forward over your right leg and clasp your foot with both hands, at the same time turning your right shoulder downwards towards your right leg and letting your left shoulder come up. Your head should be between your arms. Breathe slowly and deeply. Sit up slowly and do the same thing bending to the other side. After a breathing pause repeat once more and then rest on your back (savasana).

(Increases will-power.)

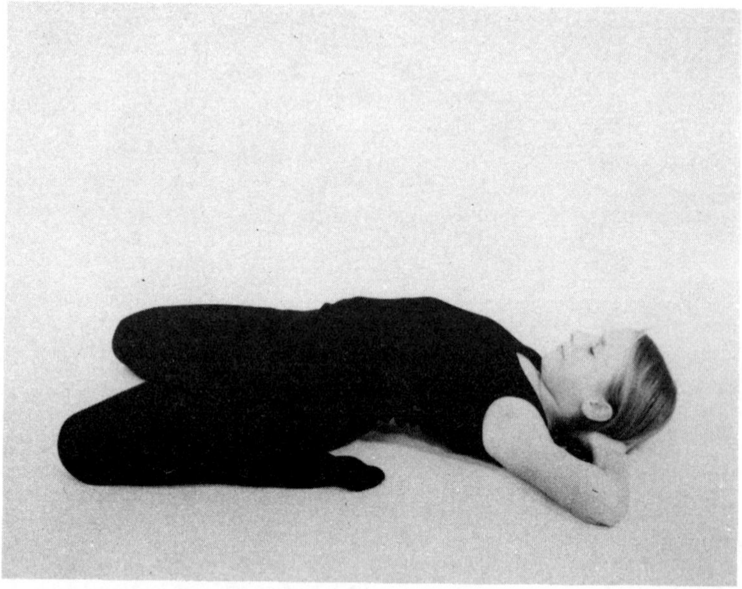

SUPTA-VADSHRASANA

Sit between your heels. Using your elbows to help you, lie back on the floor and place your hands under your neck. Breathe gently and hold the position for as long as you can without it becoming a strain. Afterwards rest on your back (savasana).

(Activates the nervous system; encourages glandular activity.)

NB: Not for anyone with an over-active thyroid gland.

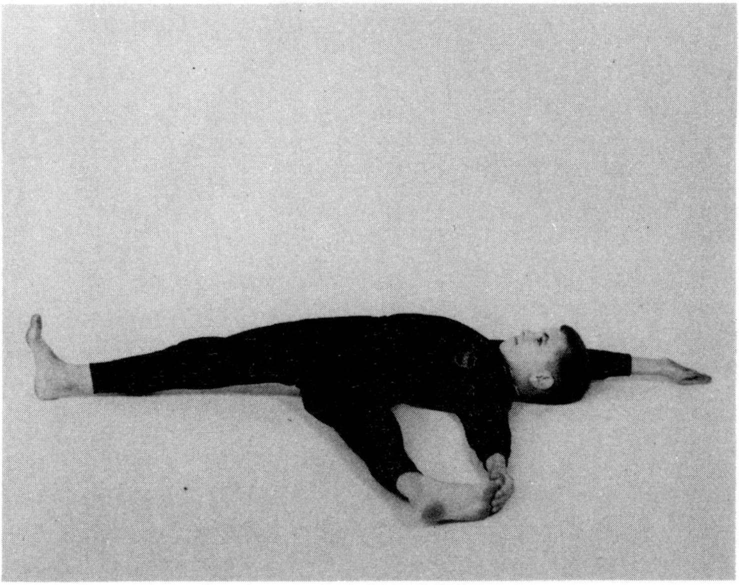

GOKARNASANA

Lie on your back with your left arm stretched out on the floor behind your head. Hold the toes of your right foot with your right hand and stretch your right leg out to the side so that it forms a right-angle to both your body and your left leg (and make sure that your knees are completely straight). Hold the position for about 20 seconds breathing deeply and regularly. Then let go of your right foot and return to your original position. Then do the same thing but on your other side. After a breathing pause, repeat the whole exercise twice then rest on your back (savasana).

(Increases physical sensitivity.)

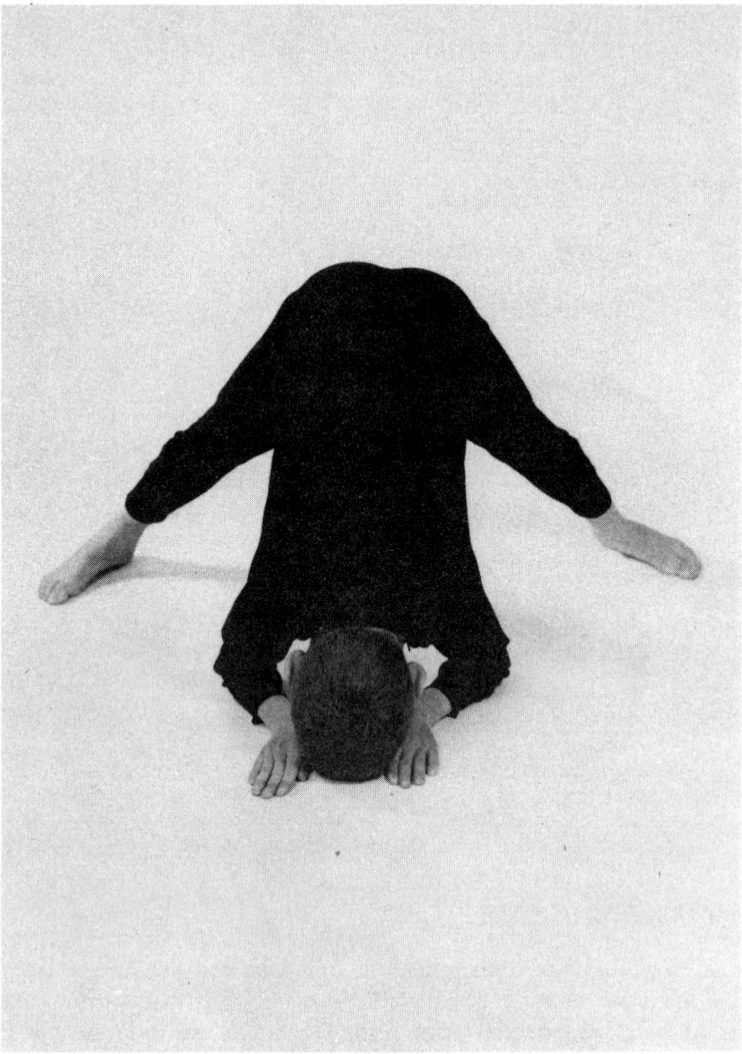

Stand with your feet apart. Bend forward and place your hands, forearms and forehead on the floor. Hold the position for a short time, then slowly stand up. After a breathing pause, repeat once, then rest on your back (savasana).

(Strengthens the back and increases flexibility.)

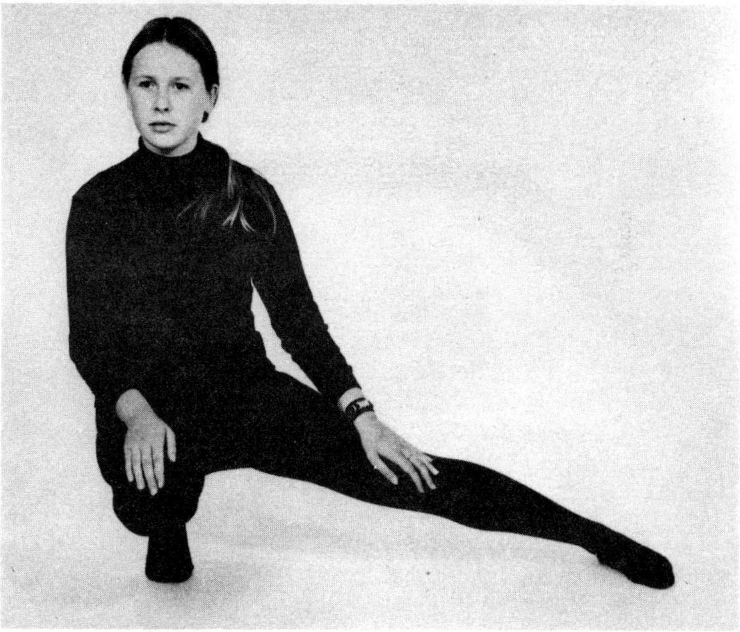

Sit in a squatting position and stretch your left leg out to the side. Keep your hands on your knees and your back straight. Transfer your weight to your left leg, stretch your right leg out and squat on your left foot. Remain in a squatting position as you transfer your weight from one foot to the other. Repeat once and then rest on your back (savasana).

(Strengthens the leg muscles).

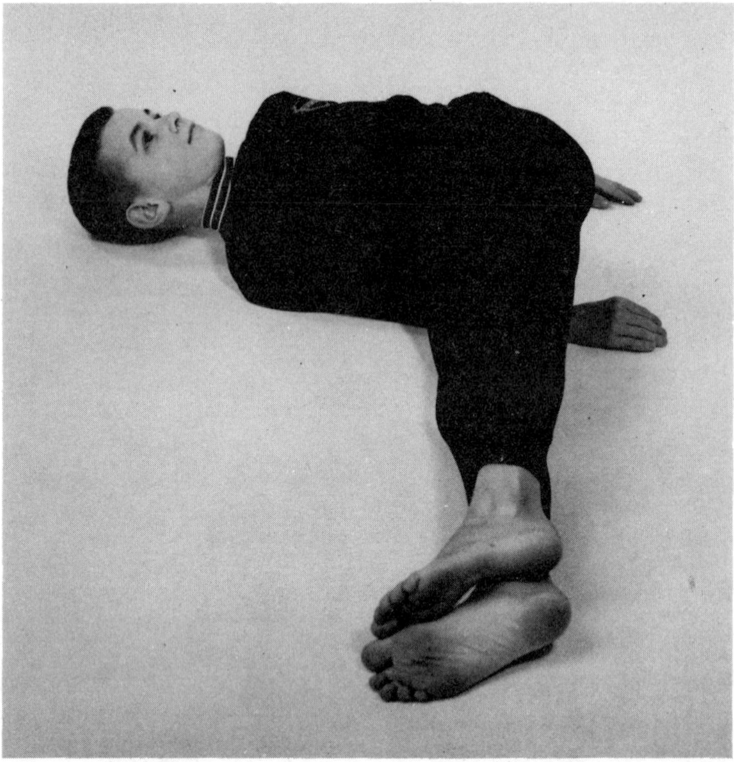

PASHVA-PADAKALANASANA (*twisting exercise*)

Lie on your back, your arms stretched out by your sides and your palms facing downwards. Breathing in, raise both legs so your toes are pointing towards the ceiling, and breathing out, bring them down to the floor on your left side. Breathing in, raise them again, and breathing out, bring them down on your right side. Breathing in, raise them once more, and breathing out, lower them and return to your original position. After a breathing pause, repeat twice and then rest on your back (savasana).

(Strengthens the abdominal and leg muscles and increases determination.)

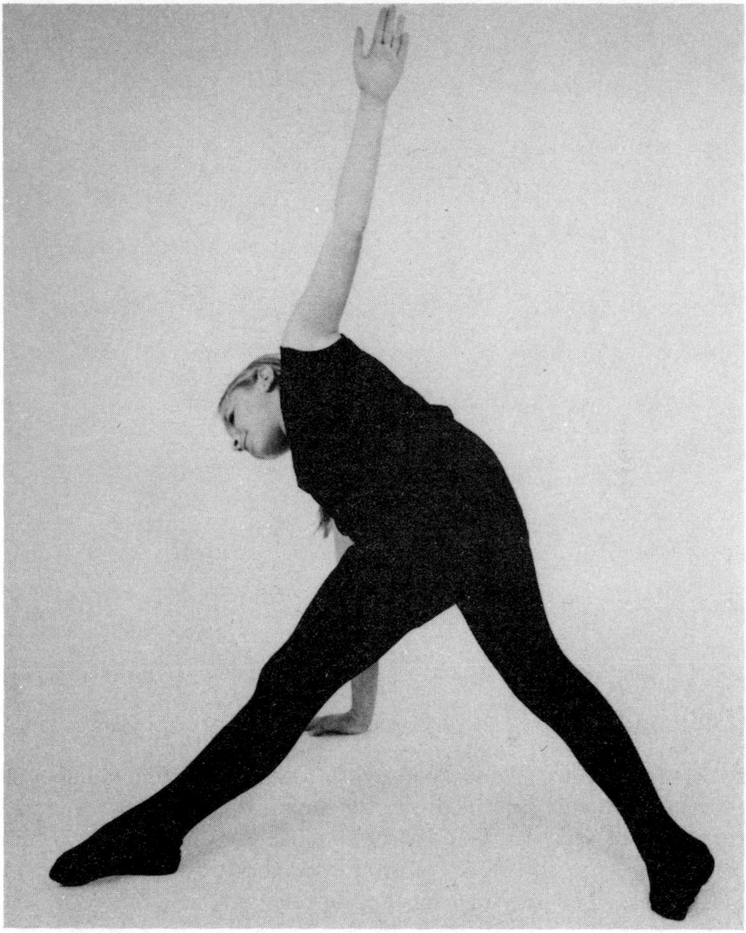

Twisting exercise

Sit with your legs wide apart, your right arm stretched out behind you for support and your left hand on your knee. Raise your left arm and shifting your weight to the right, twist your body from the waist to the right. Breathing in, raise the small of your back off the floor. Breathing out, twist back so you are facing forward, support yourself with your left arm on the floor and sit down again. Do the same on the other side and then rest on your back (savasana).

(Strengthens the spine.)

Twisting exercise

Sit with your legs wide apart, your arms stretched behind you with your hands on the floor for support. Breathing in, raise the small of your back and your left hand from the floor. Shift your weight to the right, twisting your body from the waist as far to the right as you can and support yourself on your left arm. Breathing in, lift your left arm from the floor, twist your body from the waist back to the centre so you are facing straight ahead again, and still keeping your body off the floor support it once more with your left arm. Now lift your right hand from the floor, twist your body to the left and support yourself on your right arm. Breathing in, lift your right hand from the floor and twist your body back to the centre. Supporting yourself on your right arm again, breathe out and sit down. Lay your head on your knee and breathe peacefully. After a short breathing pause, repeat the exercise on each side once more and then rest on your back (savasana).

(Strengthens the spine.)

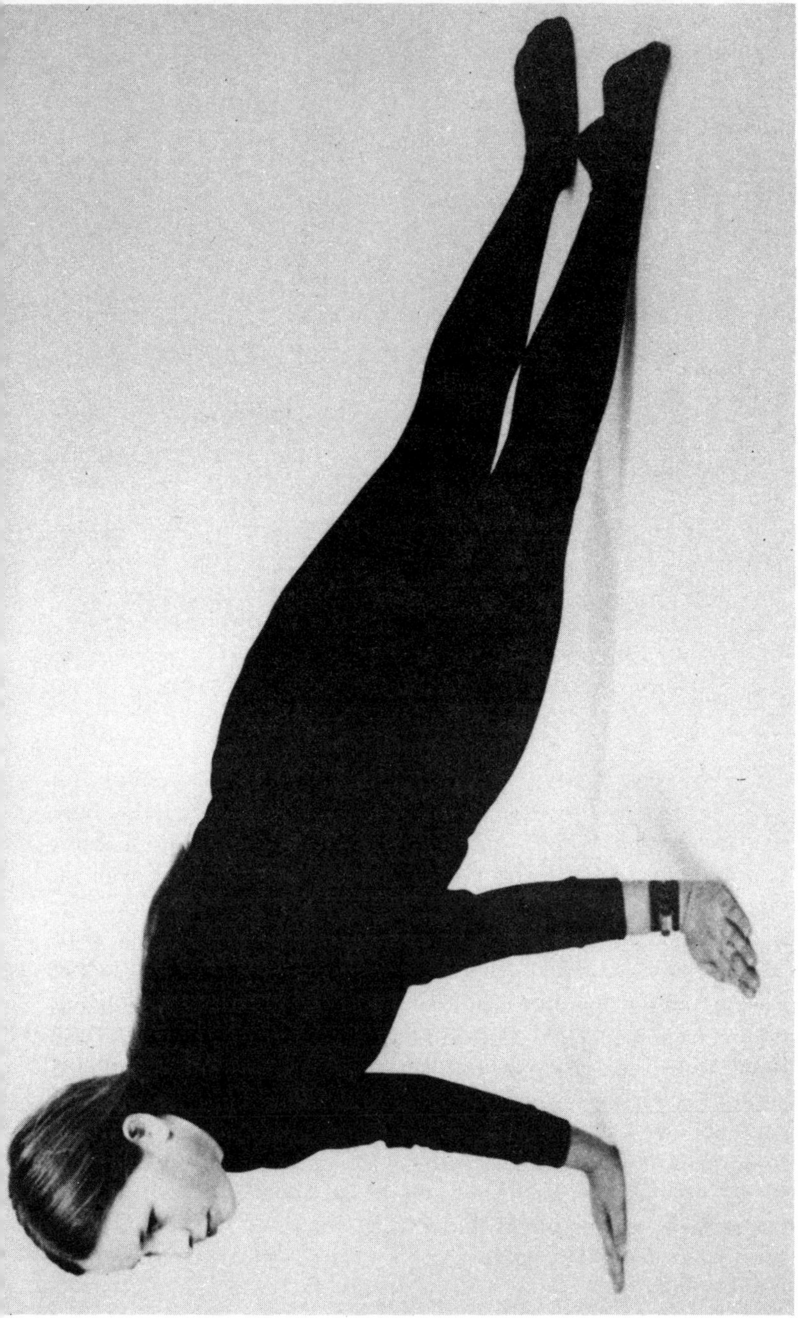

Lie on your front with your toes curled under and your hands under your shoulders. Breathing in, raise your body from the floor; make sure that you don't bend your back so that as far as possible your body remains in a straight line. Breathing out, raise your pelvis as high as you can so that your body is bent almost at a right angle. Breathing in, lower your pelvis, and breathing out, return to your original position lying on your stomach. Lay your hands under your forehead and rest. After a brief pause repeat and then rest on your back (savasana).

(Strengthens the spine.)

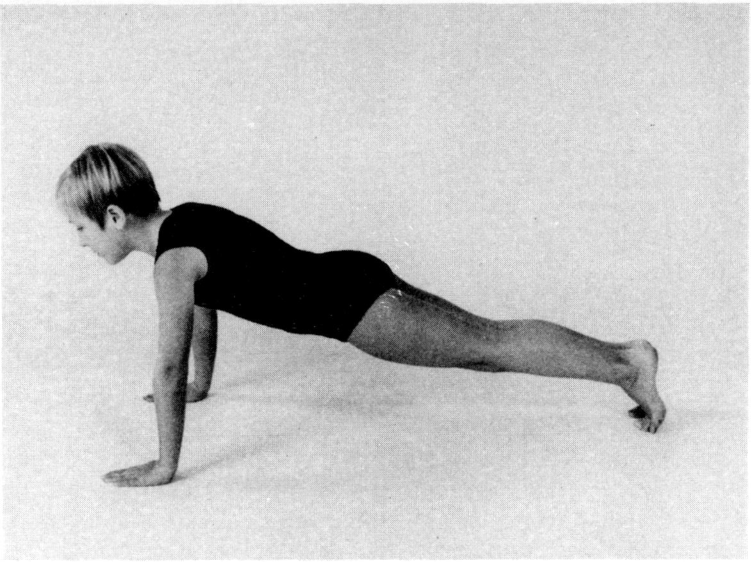

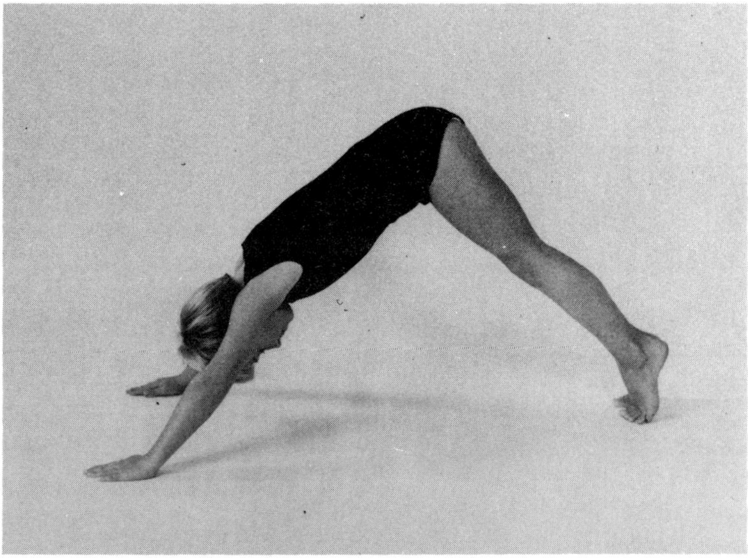

CHAKRASANA

Lie on your back, your legs bent, your feet on the floor, wide apart and close to your body. Raise your arms and place your hands under your shoulders. Breathing in deeply, raise your whole body like a bridge. Breathe slowly and deeply for a few seconds and then lie flat on your back and rest in the savasana position. You can repeat this exercise twice.

(Teaches perfect control of the spine.)

NB: Not for anyone with an over-active thyroid gland.

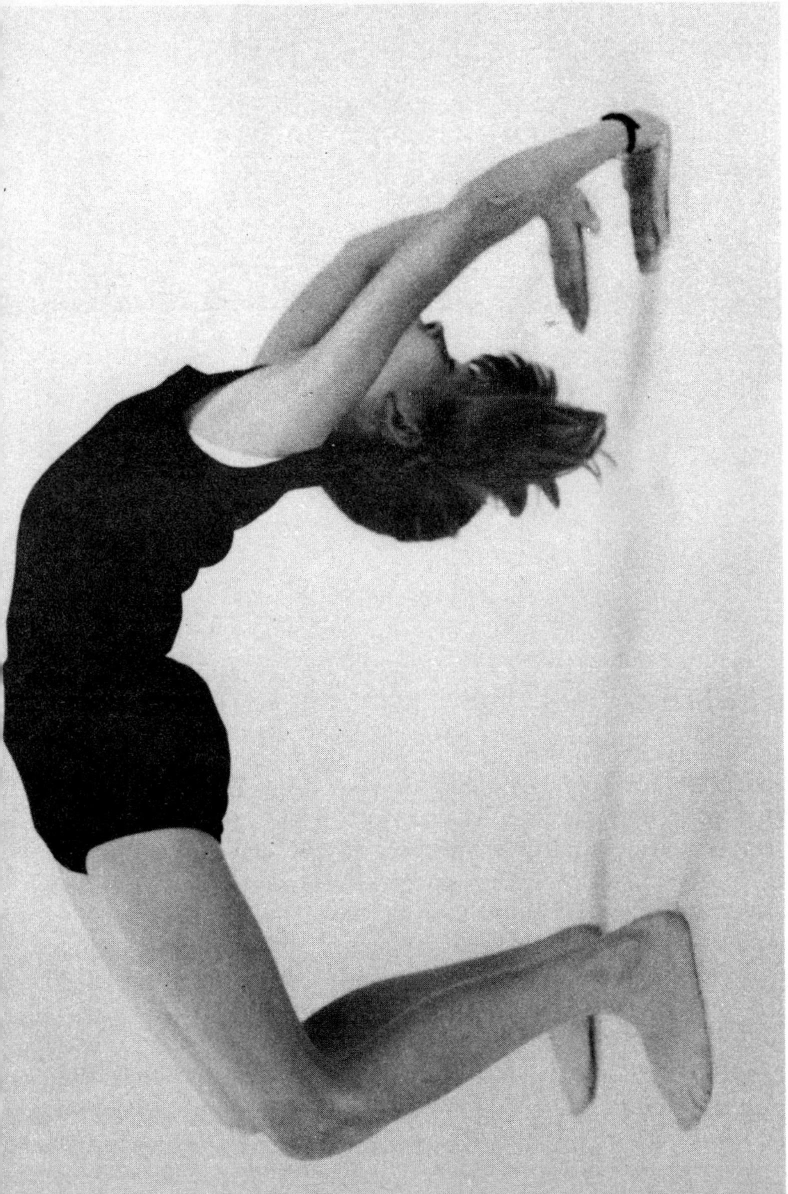

DHRITYASANA

1. Sit between your heels with both your knees and feet wide apart. Hold on to your ankles or your heels. Breathing deeply raise your body as high as you can off the ground. Hold the position for a short time breathing deeply and peacefully. Let go of your heels or ankles, straighten up, close your knees and feet together, sit on your heels and bend forward. Rest in this position with your forehead supported on your fists. Repeat twice, then rest on your back (savasana).

2. Kneel on the floor with your knees and feet apart, your back straight and your shoulders drawn back; your arms should hang loosely and relaxed. Breathe in deeply and peacefully. Breathing out, relax and bend your body backwards with your hands on your heels. Breathing in, straighten up and breathe peacefully. After a breathing pause, repeat twice, then rest on your back (savasana).

(Exercise for strengthening the abdomen, pelvis and small of the back; relieves tiredness in the small of the back.)

NB: Not for anyone with an over-active thyroid gland.

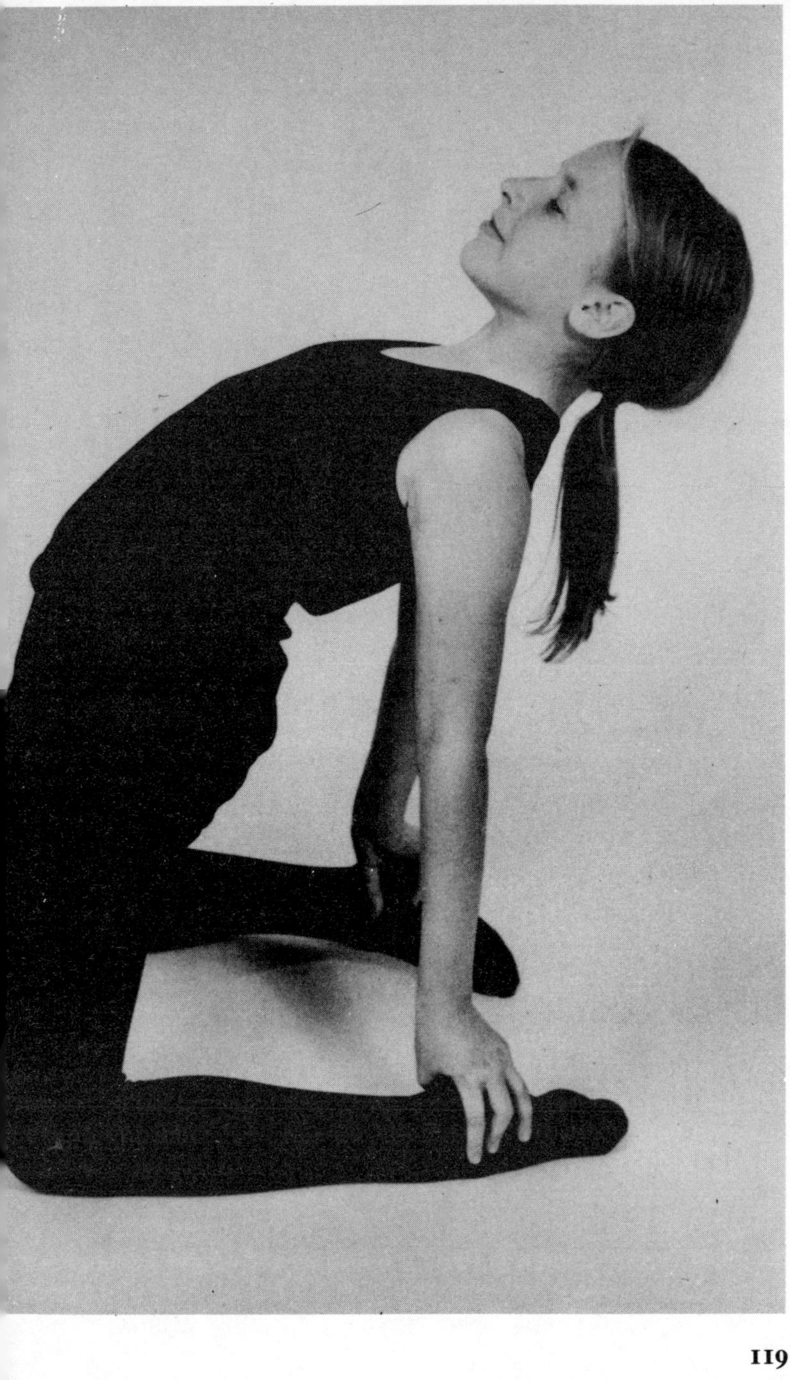

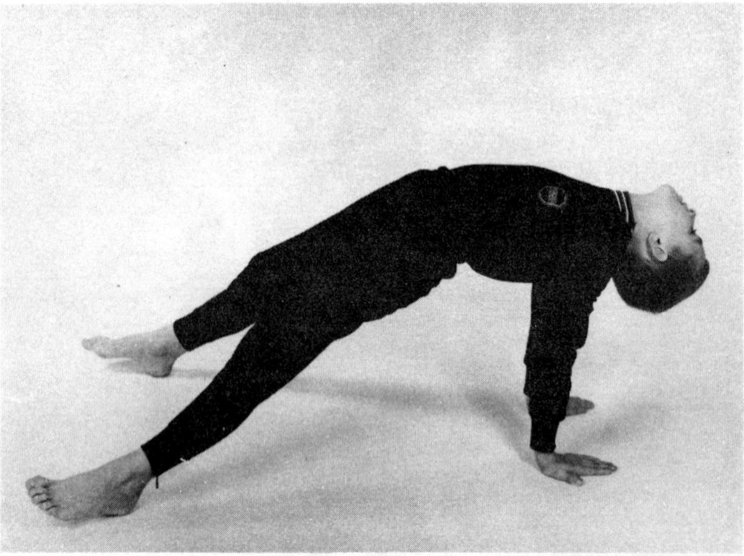

KATIKASANA

Sit with your legs wide apart, your hands on the floor behind you for support. Breathing in, slowly and cautiously raise your pelvis and the small of your back as high off the floor as you can; breathing out, lower them again. After a breathing pause, repeat twice then draw your knees up to your body and, hugging them, rest your forehead on them.

(Invigorates the spine and pelvis.)

NB: Not for anyone with an over-active thyroid gland.

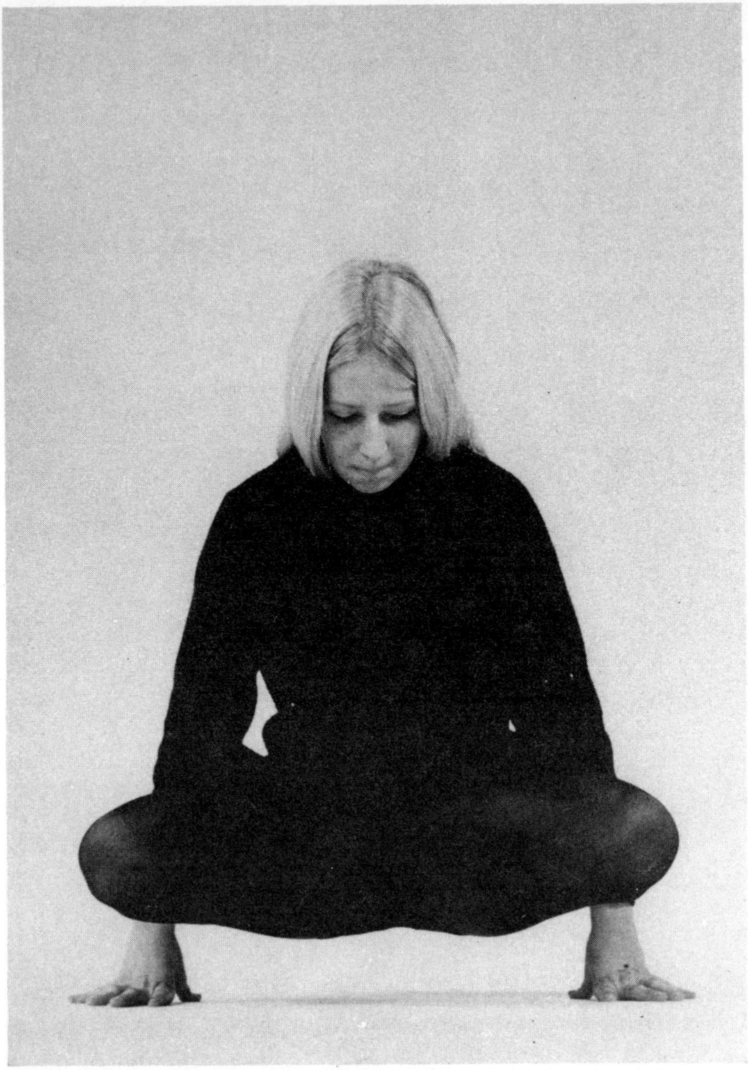

When you can sit in the lotus position without difficulty you can cautiously try to lift yourself up on your hands. Be patient and don't strain yourself.